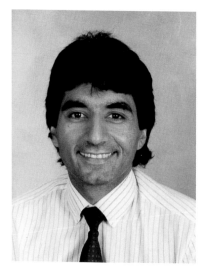
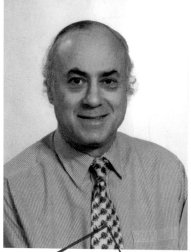

Tariq I. Mughal *(above left)*
Dr Mughal graduated from St George's Hospital Medical School,
London, UK, received postgraduate training at the University of
Colorado School of Medicine, Denver, USA and the Royal
Postgraduate Medical School, Hammersmith Hospital, London,
UK. He is a Consultant Haematologist and Medical Oncologist at
the Royal Preston Hospital, Preston and the Christie Hospital,
Manchester, UK and an Hon. Senior Lecturer at the University of
Manchester, UK.

John M. Goldman *(above right)*
Professor Goldman graduated from Oxford University, received
postgraduate training at the Massachusetts General Hospital,
Boston, USA and the Royal Postgraduate Medical School,
Hammersmith Hospital, London, UK. He is a Professor of
Leukaemia Biology at the Imperial College School of Medicine,
London, a Consultant Physician and Chairman of the Depart-
ment of Haematology at the Hammersmith Hospital, London,
UK.

Understanding Leukaemia and Related Cancers

Tariq I. Mughal
& John M. Goldman

Forewords by
José Carreras & Ray Powles

**Blackwell
Science**

© 1999 by
Blackwell Science Ltd
Editorial Offices:
Osney Mead, Oxford OX2 OEL
25 John Street, London WC1N 2BL
23 Ainslie Place, Edinburgh EH3 6AJ
350 Main Street, Malden
  MA 02148 5018, USA
54 University Street, Carlton
  Victoria 3053, Australia
10, rue Casimir Delavigne
  75006 Paris, France

Other Editorial Offices:
Blackwell Wissenschafts-Verlag GmbH
Kurfürstendamm 57
10707 Berlin, Germany

Blackwell Science KK
MG Kodenmacho Building
7–10 Kodenmacho Nihombashi
Chuo-ku, Tokyo 104, Japan

The right of the Authors to be
identified as the Authors of this Work
has been asserted in accordance
with the Copyright, Designs and
Patents Act 1988.

First published 1999

Set by Sparks Computer Solutions, Oxford
Printed and bound in Great Britain at the
University Press, Cambridge

DISTRIBUTORS

Marston Book Services Ltd
PO Box 269
Abingdon, Oxon OX14 4YN
(Orders: Tel: 01235 465500
        Fax: 01235 465555)
USA
Blackwell Science, Inc.
Commerce Place
350 Main Street
Malden, MA 02148 5018
(Orders: Tel: 800 759 6102
                781 388 8250
        Fax: 781 388 8255)
Canada
Login Brothers Book Company
324 Saulteaux Crescent
Winnipeg, Manitoba R3J 3T2
(Orders: Tel: 204 837 2987)
Australia
Blackwell Science Pty Ltd
54 University Street
Carlton, Victoria 3053
(Orders: Tel: 3 9347 0300
        Fax: 3 9347 5001)

Catalogue records for this title
are available from the British Library
and the Library of Congress

ISBN 0-632-05346-1

For further information on
Blackwell Science, visit our website:
www.blackwell-science.com

The Blackwell Science logo is a
trade mark of Blackwell Science Ltd,
registered at the United Kingdom
Trade Marks Registry

Contents

Foreword

by José Carreras

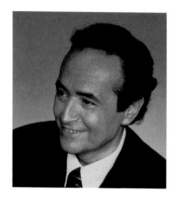

José Carreras, President,
International José Carreras
Foundation, Barcelona, Spain.

I appreciate the authors' kind invitation to write the non-medical foreword to *Understanding Leukaemia and Related Cancers*. It provides me an opportunity to communicate with patients and the public to whom I would like to bring a message of hope.

Undoubtedly the diagnosis of blood cancer irrevocably changes the lifestyle of the patient as well as the whole family. The diagnosis often carries an undercurrent of dread and even terror, largely because of the general public's perception of these diseases, much of which stems from non-medical media reports. But the medical facts speak for themselves: an increasing proportion of patients with certain types of blood cancers are now being cured. Perhaps I, myself, can be considered fortunate enough to be among them.

The authors of this book have had extensive experience in the treatment of blood cancers and have put together an enormous amount of highly technical and up-to-date information in non-technical language. The authors hide nothing, but they convey the message that the world-wide effort devoted to the study and treatment of these diseases will continue to improve the prospects of patients everywhere. Science and medicine, however, must be accompanied by a positive attitude. It takes a lot of courage from the patient and the loving support of family and friends to overcome the many hurdles posed by these diseases.

Reading *Understanding Leukaemia and Related Cancers* should facilitate a better understanding and help patients to improve their chances of cure. Knowing what lies ahead at each moment is also an important source of encouragement. Many times, the prospects of an invasive therapy, or an aggressive treatment may be devastating. The directness of the doctor–patient relationship can sometimes bring difficult episodes in the course of the curative process. However, proper information, with no false expectations but, most importantly, no unjustified fears is a crucial element in helping patients and their families. The authors' openness should provide decisive support to individuals needing to face their illness with renewed courage.

Finally, let me share with you what I recall as being the fundamental source of strength in my recovery; even if there is only a small chance of survival, that particular chance is yours and the one you fight for.

Foreword
by Professor Ray Powles

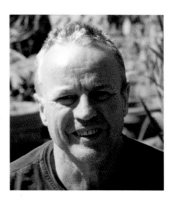

Professor Ray Powles, Head of
Adult Leukaemia Unit, Royal
Marsden Hospital, Surrey, UK.

In Chapter 5 of this book, it says 'The news usually comes as a bombshell to both the patients and relatives.' This sums up rather nicely the reason why—in my medical student days at the beginning of the 1960s—we found it so difficult to tell patients that they had leukaemia. The average survival for acute myeloid leukaemia was then 6 weeks. At that time, St Bartholomew's Hospital, London was one of the few specialist institutions in the world attempting to treat these patients. *Sir Ronald Bodley Scott*, the Queen's physician, led the team and soon after the extraordinary dynamic *Gordon Hamilton-Fairley* (subsequently killed by an IRA bomb) became his Chief Assistant. A group of young doctors were then drawn in (including one of the authors), with all the dynamic, blind optimism of youth. They were inspired to join in the race to change things; and so the modern era of leukaemia treatment was born. At that time there were two 30 bedded open-plan Nightingale Wards (male and female) at St Bartholomew's Hospital and one could always find patient outliers scattered throughout the hospital. More than a thousand patients were seen during that decade and all but a handful died. This was the background at this time, and so it was not surprising the policy in so many hospitals about telling patients was 'don't tell them the diagnosis, they will never cope with it'—when what was really meant was 'don't tell them, because none of us will cope'. The doctors often just described the patient's illness by its symptoms, saying that they had, for example, a difficult infection (which was, of course, a common cause of death for parents and grandparents of many of these patients). A book such as this one was a million miles from anybody's dreams. How times have changed in my working lifetime!

Since the 1960s there has been an explosion of technology and understanding of leukaemia—described well in these pages—in which the subtle diagnosis of the various forms of leukaemia has been reduced to the molecular level, so that we now know the sequence of the genetic code involved (this disease is not inherited) and how it has changed. This had led to a large, tailor-made portfolio of effective treatments often given as modules in sequence with cure expectancies of up to 70% for good-risk acute leukaemia. A second and third generation of doctors, scientists, and other health care workers has learned by experience, research and trials information on an exponential scale and, with modern technology, this information is now easily handled.

Crucially, the patients now not only have expectations of success but also with the advent of patient education they have the right and need to know what is happening to them. This information is essential for them to understand and be involved in decisions and give informed consent to their management. Exact knowledge of their condition has been a great help to many patients in that they can now visualize in their own minds their disease and what they are fighting against, and create the environment of positive thinking which is so important to quality of life and outcome.

Many patients want to know what caused their disease and this book nicely and precisely defines what is known on this subject. However, it rightly devotes only a relatively small amount of space to this subject because it is unlikely in the foreseeable (and perhaps even distant) future that we will be able to prevent leukaemia. Therefore, once it has already developed in a patient it can be very negative to dwell too much on the cause, with all the unproductive emotions of anger, bewilderment, guilt, etc., particularly with such effective treatments now available. The authors of this book want patients to look forward and face the future positively and therefore they balance nicely the essential facts relating to cause and treatment that patients need to know, so they tackle their problems in the journey to come. Details relating to treatment are important because each patient is different, often facing a sequence of many varying drug and transplant schedules. It is assumed that patients and relatives really want to know most about their own particular disease and its treatment and we know that each patient's coping mechanism is different, so this book is structured so that it can be used easily by patients and their relatives for specific bits of information. Some patients (a good example are doctors with leukaemia) often find it far too stressful to know any specific details of prognosis and treatment other than practicalities, e.g. 'When will I get out of the hospital?' Many others will also want only specific information, such as details of support groups found in this book, or access to the remarkably comprehensive glossary so that key words can be looked up before and after interviews with health care workers. It is likely that relatives of patients will find this particularly helpful, because, in general, they take in so much more about what is being discussed, particularly in the very frightening early period after diagnosis.

This book is wonderfully positive throughout, so full of energy, and justifiably optimistic. In the most part, it is gently and kindly worded and not defensive, patronising or, as is the nature of standard textbooks, brutal. It reflects hopefully the more approachable, less-aloof changes in the perception by patients of health care workers, especially doctors. Approachability and ever improving communication skills are now mandatory, and this book acts as an index of our concern within the profession to be ever vigilant in increasing our awareness of our patient's emotional and physical plight during this stressful, sometimes painful and often depressing period in their lives. We wish every one of them success and a return to normal life.

Authors' note

This book is intended for a varied audience, including patients and their families, nonspecialist doctors, medical students and health workers. We have therefore had to walk a narrow path, avoiding, on the one hand, confusing medical jargon and unwarranted assumptions about the level of familiarity of the reader and, on the other hand, over-simplification. We have endeavoured not to sacrifice scientific accuracy for clarity, or vice versa.

Some patients or their families may find our detailed descriptions of treatment excessive, cold and clinical, but we believe that most will benefit from understanding not only what is being done but also why it is being done. This is in keeping with the modern view that patients (and/or their families) should be participants in their medical care.

Acknowledgements

We would like to thank Dr David B. Lewall, Professor Andrew Padmos, Professor Howie Scarfe, Professor Miltiadias Stefadouros, Mr Jack Tressidder, and many friends for reading the various draft manuscripts and the final version of this book and for diligently discussing its contents. We also wish to thank Professor David Galton and Professor Derek Crowther for their guidance, Sabena Mughal for the original cover suggestion, and Miss Ma. Sofia Claridad and Mrs Kate Harding for typing the manuscript and Mr Paul Chantry for the art work. T. M. also wishes to thank his daughter Sabena for the loving attention, comments (and tolerance) expressed during the preparation of this book.

1 What is leukaemia?

Introduction

Put very simply, leukaemia is cancer of the blood, and in order to understand it, it is helpful to know something about both the history of cancer and the nature of cancer in general.

Cancer is not new to the twentieth century; it has been recognised for more than 2000 years. Even the earliest medical scientists such as Hippocrates, Galen and Paracelsus knew about cancer. They described it as a 'crab-like' uncontrolled growth (hence the name). They also recognised that these growths (called tumours) could arise from most organs of the body, that they could grow to interfere with the normal functioning of the affected organ and that they could spread to other parts of the body where they could do further damage, which would eventually lead to death. What these early pioneers did not know, and what is still largely a mystery even today, is why tumours start and why they grow in such characteristic ways.

One reason why cancer seems more common today may be simply that more people are living long enough to suffer from it. Until very recently infectious diseases were a major cause of death before late middle age, which is when cancer usually appears. In the days before antibiotics, even a simple bacterial infection of a finger or toe could lead to septicaemia (blood poisoning) and death. Only a hundred years ago, very many children and young adults died of infections such as pneumonia, meningitis, smallpox and diphtheria; these diseases have now been virtually eliminated in most parts of the developed world, though they are still frequent in some parts of the world.

In developed countries, most deaths are now related to degeneration (sometimes called hardening) of the arteries in which the blood vessels that supply blood to the heart or brain gradually become narrower, eventually leading to heart attacks and strokes. Almost three-quarters of the people alive today will die of either heart or brain blood vessel problems. Of the remainder, most will die as a result of cancer.

As mentioned above, leukaemia is cancer of the blood. The term itself was first used over a century ago by a German physician called Virchow, who observed that some patients seemed to be affected by a condition leading to 'weisses blut' (German for 'white blood', later translated into Greek as λευχαιμια 'leukaemia'). The term 'white blood' was used because at that time it was thought that the high number of white blood cells in the blood actually made the blood appear to be white. Although this was later shown to be untrue, the term 'leukaemia' continued to be used to describe this disease.

What happens in cancer?

Cancer affects a population of cells in the body and it is therefore necessary to know something about cells in order to un-

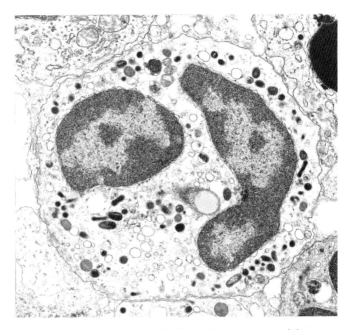

Figure 1.1 A normal white blood cell, in this case a neutrophil, magnified 16 000 times by an electron microscope. (Courtesy of Dr Brian Eyden, Christie Hospital, Manchester, UK.)

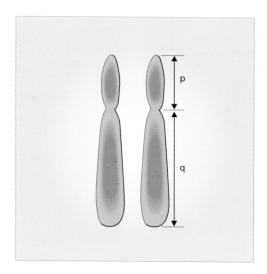

Figure 1.2 A schematic diagram of a human chromosome.

derstand what happens in cancer. Cells are the tiny living components which make up the body. They are usually so small that they cannot be seen unless they are magnified at least 100 times with a microscope. Figure 1.1 is a picture of a cell which has been magnified 16 000 times by an electron microscope. There are many different types of cells but they all have a surface membrane (like the skin of a peach), cytoplasm (like the pulp), and a nucleus (the pip), which can be thought of as the cell's brain.

We all begin life as a single cell that divides and whose progeny divide, over and over, according to a unique set of coded instructions present in its nucleus. Each set consists of many parts called genes. Currently it is believed that we have over 90 000 genes in each cell. Within each nucleus rows of genes are arranged in strings, known as chromosomes. A gene can therefore be considered as a tiny part of a chromosome. The human chromosome is a complex structure made up of genes and several different proteins. Chromosomes, which are present in all cells, pass on information about the cell's functions to its offspring. During the process of normal cell division and duplication, each chromosome has to be duplicated. Each chromosome has two arms (see Fig. 1.2), a short arm known as 'p' (for petit) and a long arm known as 'q' (the

3

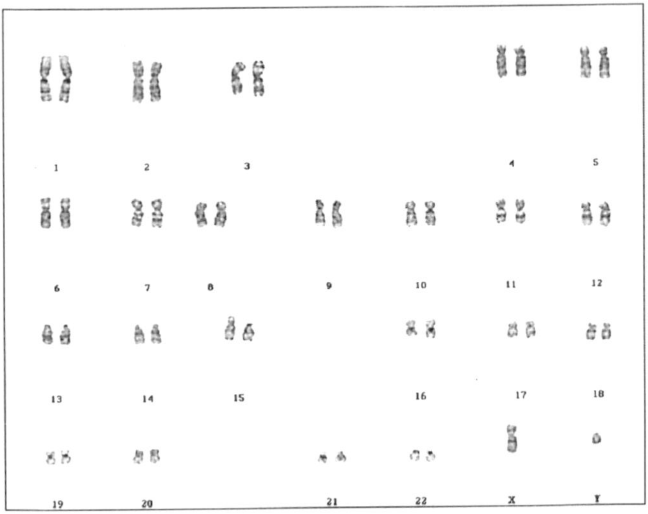

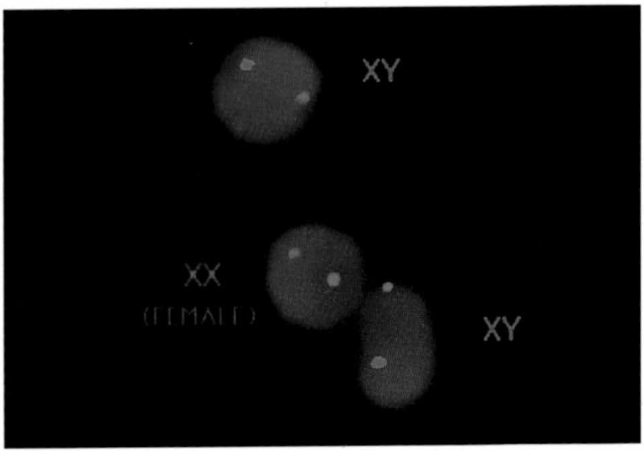

Figure 1.3 A photomicrograph of normal human male and female karyotypes. (Courtesy of Ms Una Maye, Christie Hospital, Manchester, UK.)

letter after 'p' in the alphabet). A normal human cell contains 23 pairs of chromosomes, including a pair of so-called sex chromosomes; in the female both sex chromosomes are designated X, while in the male, one is designated X and one Y. Chromosomes vary in size with the longest being the chromosome designated number 1. Each complete set of chromosomes is called a karyotype. The normal female karyotype is described as 46, XX and the male 46, XY. Figure 1.3 is a photomicrographic representation of normal human male and female karyotypes.

Each gene consists of a substance known as deoxyribonucleic acid (DNA), and it is the DNA which determines exactly how our bodies are assembled and which gives us our individual characteristics. At present, scientists have been able to determine the precise DNA sequence of over 90% of the currently known human genes. This is a truly remarkable feat and it is highly probable that we should know all of the DNA sequences as early as the beginning of the next millennium. (This is a principal objective of the Human Genome Mapping Project).

When a gene is switched on, for example, by a specific message to its DNA, the cell which harbours it will respond by synthesizing a particular protein, which may subsequently cause the cell to divide. As the cells divide, they specialise. For example, the cells which make up the liver are programmed to break down the waste-products of the blood and the cells which make up the muscle of the heart are programmed to contract rhythmically in response to an electrical stimulus so that the heart is able to pump blood through our body.

Our body is made up of some 30 trillion (3×10^{13}) cells. Unless they need to be mobile, all cells with the same function cluster together to form an organ. When several organs have related functions, they also work together, as organ systems. For instance, the respiratory organ system consists of the nose, mouth, windpipe and lungs, which all work together to provide the body with oxygen. There are many such organ systems which work in cooperation under the overall control of the brain. The various organs and organ systems are linked together by blood vessels and lymphatic vessels. The blood vessels, which carry blood throughout the body, include veins, arteries and capillaries. The lymphatic vessels circulate lymph, a colourless fluid which resembles blood (but does not have red blood cells or other blood constituents), from the body tissues to the heart.

When an organ is damaged, some of the intact cells that survive may divide in order to repair the damage. Almost nothing is known about the control systems that tell a normal cell when to divide and when not to divide. The past decade has witnessed an enormous amount of research aimed at unravelling some of these mysteries. It has become clear that cells need both the ability to divide and to 'self-destruct' at the appropriate time. This may sound terribly strange and perhaps even insane! It is in fact a crucial natural process to main-

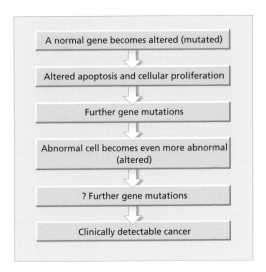

A normal gene becomes altered (mutated)

Altered apoptosis and cellular proliferation

Further gene mutations

Abnormal cell becomes even more abnormal (altered)

? Further gene mutations

Clinically detectable cancer

Figure 1.4 A schematic representation of how cancer arises.

tain the smooth and orderly functions of the body. The ability to self-destruct, often referred to as a cell suicide, is called apoptosis (αποπτωσις, a Greek word meaning literally 'dropping off'). Researchers have speculated that a breakdown in the systems which control cell division (proliferation) and facilitate apoptosis contributes to cancer. In most cases, cancer originates from a single cell that previously seemed to be completely normal, but which starts to divide in an uncontrolled way. All of the cells produced from it carry the same defect, so they also continue to divide without control. Additionally, these cells lack the ability to kill themselves and can perhaps be referred to as cells which have forgotten to die!

The modern concept of how cancer arises is shown schematically in Fig. 1.4. Despite the stark fact that there are over a hundred different varieties of cancers, the fundamental processes that result in these cancers appear to be remarkably similar. It seems that a cell becomes cancerous when an abnormality (mutation) develops in a gene. Subsequently when this gene is switched on, it will result in the production of an abnormal (mutated) protein which alters the cell's potential to divide, usually by increasing its proliferation. Most of these altered cells will remain otherwise indistinguishable from their normal counterparts. Following a variable period, ranging from a few months to several years, further mutations occur within the altered gene. This results in a further change in the cell's growth, often resulting in an abnormal appearance. Many such abnormal cells remain 'contained' by the body's defence mechanisms, but ultimately they may acquire additional abnormalities, usually as a consequence of further gene mutations, and it then becomes apparent to the clinician that they are cancerous. Scientists have discovered an enzyme called telomerase, which is an essential component of the body's control system that prevents cells from continuing to multiply out of control. In the next paragraph we will discuss some of the recent advances which have provided important clues to the underlying processes leading to gene mutations, as we focus on how leukaemias arise—a process referred to as leukaemogenesis.

The growing lump of cells (the tumour) not only disturbs the normal function of the organ in which it started, but it can also invade surrounding organs. For example, a tumour that starts in the uterus (womb) may grow to affect the inner wall of the pelvis. Portions of the parent tumour can also escape from the main bulk and travel via the blood or lymphatic vessels to other sites in the body. This process is referred to as 'metastasis', from the Greek μεθιστασθαι 'a migration'. Once at the new site, the cancer cells can grow and cause a new tumour, also referred to as a metastasis. Occasionally, a metastasis will be mistaken as the primary tumour if, for some reason, the parent tumour has escaped detection.

As mentioned earlier there are many forms of cancer. The most common form of cancers are carcinomas (καρκινος, from the Greek word meaning 'crab-like'). Carcinomas are cancers which arise from the epithelial tissues. Leukaemia is a cancer that starts in the bone marrow and manifests itself in the blood, so it is not a carcinoma. There are several different kinds of leukaemia. Each one is a distinct disease, affecting different age groups, requiring different forms of treatment and having different outcomes. To understand something about the different types of leukaemia, it is necessary first to have some knowledge about the components of the blood.

Components of the blood

An adult man has about 4 l of blood; women and children

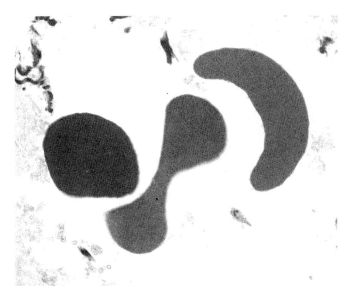

Figure 1.5 An electron micrograph showing three red blood cells magnified 12 000 times. Note that they do not have a nucleus, and that the middle red blood cell shows the typical biconcave shape. (Courtesy of Dr Brian Eyden, Christie Hospital, Manchester, UK.)

have somewhat less in proportion to their size. Blood consists of a yellow fluid, plasma, in which are suspended three major types of cells—red blood cells, white blood cells and platelets.

Red blood cells (erythrocytes) are disc-shaped with a shallow concavity on both large surfaces. Figure 1.5 shows an electron micrograph of normal red blood cells. They contain a fluid which is rich in enzymes as well as a red pigment called haemoglobin. The main function of the red blood cells is to carry inhaled oxygen from the lungs to the tissues, where it is used to release stored energy. Carbon dioxide, produced in the tissues, is carried by the red cells to the lungs, where it is exhaled from the body. There are about 5 million red blood cells in a cubic millimetre of blood. It is the great number of red blood cells that gives blood its characteristic red colour.

Far less numerous but much more specialised in their function are the white blood cells (leucocytes). Each cubic millimetre of blood contains only about 4000–10 000 leucocytes. There are three major types of leucocytes—granulocytes, monocytes and lymphocytes. All three are important compo-

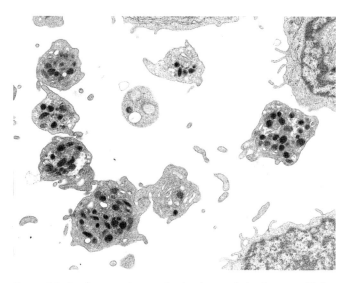

Figure 1.6 An electron micrograph of a cluster of platelets magnified 13 000 times. (Courtesy of Dr Brian Eyden, Christie Hospital, Manchester, UK.)

nents of the immune system and help in fighting infection and in destroying alien material within the body. The granulocytes and the monocytes work by ingesting unwanted particles such as bacteria or fungi and then destroying them by releasing destructive enzymes contained within their granules. Lymphocytes can recognise bacteria and viruses and then divide to form more lymphocytes which secrete a variety of substances that may destroy the invaders. Alternatively, they may recruit other white blood cells to help. These helper cells are called T-lymphocytes because they come from the *thymus* gland, an organ found behind the breastbone (sternum). Other types of white blood cells, referred to as B-lymphocytes (because they were first discovered in an organ called the *bursa*— the chicken equivalent of the human bone marrow), secrete proteins (antibodies) that can interact with and destroy bacteria and viruses in the body.

The third type of cell in the blood is the platelet or thrombocyte. Figure 1.6 shows an electron micrograph of a normal

Figure 1.7 Normal development of blood cells (haemopoiesis). *(Overleaf.)*

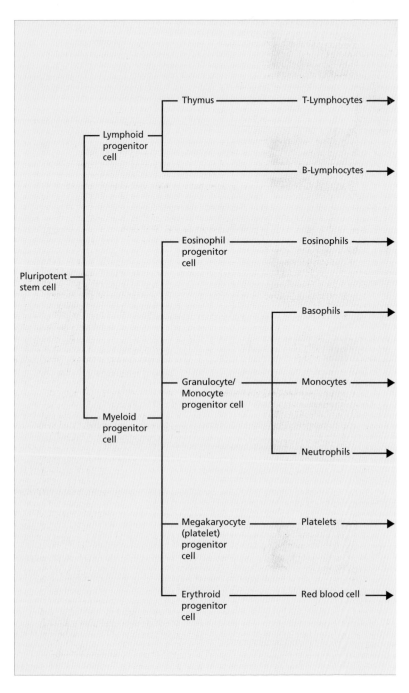

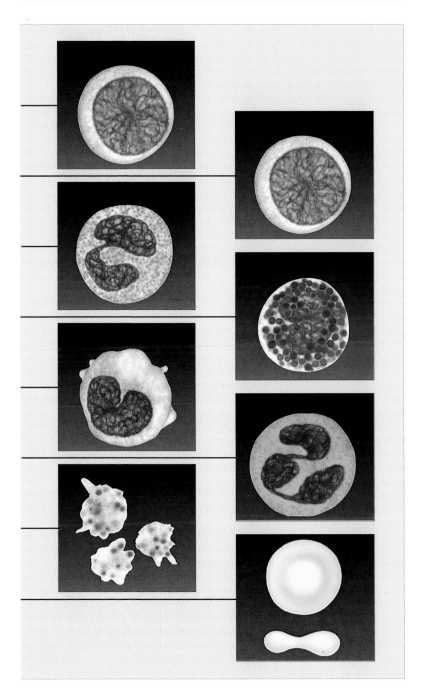

platelet. The main functions of these tiny cells are to clump together to plug small holes in blood vessels, and to release the chemical necessary to start and maintain blood clotting. Platelets are therefore vital in the maintenance of small blood vessels, and spontaneous bleeding may occur if there are too few of them. Normally, there are about 150–400 thousand platelets in a cubic millimetre of blood.

Unlike many other cells in the body, the population of blood cells is not fixed; blood cells are released into the blood where they circulate until they die. Red blood cells survive in the bloodstream for about 120 days and are continuously replaced. The life span of white blood cells is variable, ranging from only a few hours (some granulocytes) to months or years (some lymphocytes). Platelets survive for 4–8 days.

After birth, all blood cells are made in the bone marrow and are released into the bloodstream. In adults, marrow fills the cavities of all the major bones. The bones of the pelvis and vertebral column, the ribs, breastbone and, to a lesser extent, the upper arm and upper leg consist of an outer layer of thick, hard bone, the cortex; inside there is spongy bone, the cavities of which are filled with marrow.

To the naked eye, bone marrow looks like jelly, but under the microscope it can be seen to consist of fat cells interspersed with cells that will eventually become blood cells, all in various stages of development. Although mature red blood cells, white blood cells and platelets are also present in the marrow, most marrow cells are stem cells, the parents and grandparents of blood cells, which maintain blood production, or haemopoiesis (see Fig. 1.7). The development from stem cell to the release of the mature red blood cell, white blood cell or platelet into the bloodstream takes about 10–14 days.

When a defect causes too few blood cells to be produced or when there is something wrong with the blood cells, problems arise. If it is mainly the red blood cells that are affected, the patient will appear pale or anaemic. The tissues will not receive enough oxygen, and this will make the patient feel tired and weak. If white blood cells are affected, the body's ability to fight germs will be impaired and the patient will be more likely to get infections. If platelets are involved, there will be a tendency for bruising and bleeding, primarily from the gums or nose. Sometimes small blood vessels will leak and produce tiny skin bleeds, called 'petechiae', which resemble freckles.

Progress in understanding the blood has been closely linked to the development of improved techniques for examining both it and the bone marrow. The introduction of microscopes capable of magnifying particles by 100 times or more led to the recognition of red blood cells at the end of the 18th century and of white blood cells at the beginning of the 19th century. The number of white blood cells which would normally be found in the circulation was defined soon after, and in 1845 Bennett was the first to describe patients who had an excess of white blood cells in their circulation for which no infectious or other cause could be found. Such patients were described as having 'leucocythaemia', from the Greek for white (λευκος), blood (αιμα) and cell (κυτταρον). Subsequently, the term was abbreviated to leukaemia (λευχαιμια). When the blood of patients with increased numbers of white blood cells was examined by special staining techniques, it was found that the specific white blood cell affected varied from patient to patient. This discovery led to the modern classifications of leukaemia which will be described in Chapter 3.

2 What happens in leukaemia?

It has been thought for many years that malignant cells in general and leukaemia cells in particular carry certain characteristics in their genetic make-up that are unique in that they enable genetic changes to be passed from one cell to another (horizontally; somatically) as opposed to the usual inherited changes that are carried from parent to child (vertically; germline). Why this should be so is not yet clear.

For 50 years or more it has been known that DNA, which is found in the nucleus of every mammalian cell, is the basis of both normal and abnormal genetic programming. However, only in the last 30 years have scientists begun to understand the mechanisms by which DNA is passed from a cell to its offspring, and how DNA contains a message through which it can produce another nucleic acid called messenger ribonucleic acid (mRNA) which in turn, produces a specific protein. The work of Watson and Crick at Cambridge University, UK, which was a major breakthrough in understanding this, won them a Nobel Prize in 1962. In the last 10 years scientists have begun to understand not only the molecular mechanisms that control cell division but also how these mechanisms can be subverted in the malignant cell. Some of these concepts were discussed in Chapter 1.

Oncogenes

Each cell in the body appears to have on its surface very specialised protein molecules, called receptors, which receive messages from the immediate environment and transmit them to the cell pulp (cytoplasm) and then to the cell nucleus. Certain cells produce specialised molecules that are released into the surrounding fluid and eventually make contact with appropriate receptors on other cells. Each specific molecule links only with its complementary receptor, like a key in a lock.

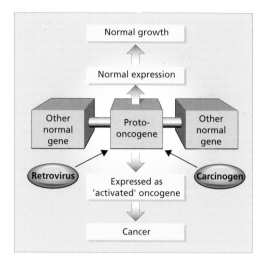

Figure 2.1 How proto-oncogenes are activated to become oncogenes.

Some of these itinerant molecules, called growth factors, are probably similar to the hormones that are produced by glands such as the thyroid or testis. Some of these growth factors travel around the body, whereas others function only in the immediate environment where they are released. Some are primarily stimulants and cause cells to divide, while others probably inhibit cell growth and division and may be thought of as retarding or suppressive substances.

In a few cases, the particular gene in normal human DNA that directs the production of a particular growth factor has been identified. When such genes are components of pathways that when disturbed lead to malignant growth, they are termed proto-oncogenes. It is important to be clear, however, that proto-oncogenes do not themselves cause cancer. On the contrary, they are present in the DNA make-up, or genome, of every normal person. Rather, proto-oncogenes are sequences of DNA that are susceptible to mutations, which then cause growth changes that include cancer. This is why, in the parlance of molecular and cell biology, genes with the potential to become cancerous oncogenes are called proto-oncogenes. Figure 2.1 depicts schematically how proto-oncogenes become oncogenes which can cause normal cells to become cancerous. The human body also possesses another class of genes called tumour suppressor genes which normally prevent the cancerous growth that would be encouraged by oncogenes. These two types of gene orchestrate the normal life span (cycle) of the altered (mutated) cell. Just as proto-oncogenes can become oncogenes when they mutate, alterations acquired by the tumour suppressor genes can also lead to cancerous growth, for example when mutations make them inactive.

In order to understand how the natural life cycle of the cells is perturbed by the acquisition of the various abnormalities in the stimulatory genes (proto-oncogenes) and inhibitory (tumour suppressor) genes, we should understand the phases through which a cell passes as it divides. The cell cycle, shown schematically in Fig. 2.2, consists of four well characterised stages (or phases). During the first stage, known as the G_1 phase (the G_1 stands for gap 1), the cell increases in size and prepares to duplicate its DNA, which will occur in the second stage, known as the S phase (the S stands for synthesis). During the S phase the cellular DNA is duplicated and a complete copy of the chromosome complement is made. The cell then enters the third stage, termed the G_2 phase (G_2 stands for gap 2) during which the cell prepares itself for division. The cell divides when it enters the fourth and final stage termed the M phase (the M stands for mitosis, from the Greek term μιτοσις

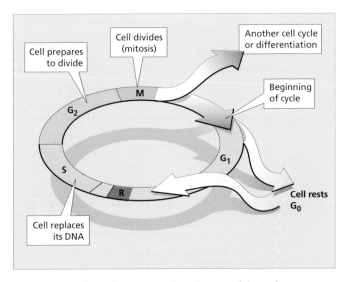

Figure 2.2 A schematic representation of stages of the cycle.

meaning division). During the M phase, each cell divides (in half) to produce two 'daughter' cells, each of which is endowed with a complete set of chromosomes. Each 'daughter cell' then usually enters the first stage (G_1) and the cycle is repeated thereafter. Alternatively, the 'daughter' cells have the option of stepping 'out of cycle' either temporarily or permanently. This phase is termed G_o, when cells rest completely.

We now know that the cell cycle clock and cancerous growth are intimately linked. Independently of the various gene mutations, it seems that the cell cycle clock can become deregulated by an alteration of the various growth factors (see above) and other proteins which are essential for an orderly and timely operation of the clock. There appear to be a number of crucial points, particularly when the cell cycle progresses from the G_1 phase to the S phase. It is here that a cell decides either to proceed further in the cycle or stop cycling (and therefore to enter the G_o phase). This 'decision point' appears to be analogous to a light switch. Scientists have now identified a series of key proteins which are involved in the operation of this switch. Two families of such proteins have been identified recently: the stimulatory proteins and the inhibitory proteins. The latter proteins, for example protein 53 (p53) and protein 16 (p16), have been implicated in the development of leukaemias. In general, when the cell cycle clock is disrupted, the cell proliferates excessively.

Apoptosis (cell suicide), which was discussed in Chapter 1, is the human body's attempt to prevent the uncontrolled proliferation of cells. Cancer cells circumvent this defence mechanism by several means. For example, p53 inhibitory protein has the ability to promote apoptosis; p53 in leukaemic cells is inactivated in chronic myeloid leukaemia (CML) so leukaemic cells fail to die off. Another protein, termed bcl-2, hinders apoptosis in patients with low grade lymphatic cancers (lymphomas).

Much of the recent cancer research in leukaemogenesis has revealed the presence of specific chromosomal abnormalities in most human leukaemias. These abnormalities serve to establish the precise location of the altered (mutated) gene. Current technology enables us to study each chromosomal breakpoint efficiently and identify the disrupted genes. The information generated is helping us to improve the treatment which will be discussed in Chapter 6.

Chromosomal alterations can be quantitative (abnormalities of numbers) or qualitative (abnormalities of structure). Numeric changes result from either a gain or loss of chromosomes; for example, loss of one number 7 chromosome, termed monosomy 7 (see Fig. 6.4), often carries a high risk for the individual to develop acute myeloid leukaemia (AML). Chromosomal translocations are the most common chromosomal alterations and result from a transfer, usually reciprocal, of genetic material between certain chromosomes. One of the best examples of this is the Philadelphia chromosome, the hallmark of chronic myeloid leukaemia (CML), which has taught us much about leukaemia cytogenetics (the area of human biology involving chromosomes). The Philadelphia chromosome, shown in Fig. 2.3, is an abnormal chromosome which usually results from a reciprocal transfer of genetic material between chromosomes number 9 and 22. We will discuss this and other well-characterised translocations associated with leukaemias in the next chapter. An interesting and currently poorly understood observation is that many chromosomal abnormalities are not unique to a particular cancer.

How prevalent is leukaemia?

Leukaemia is a relatively rare condition which is found throughout the world, although the distribution of some types varies from area to area. For example, about 2500 new cases of AML are reported each year in the USA, about 2700 in Europe, but apparently far fewer in Africa. In contrast, acute lymphoblastic leukaemia (ALL) has a relatively consistent distribution throughout the world, although different subtypes are more common in some countries than in others. The incidence of CML appears to be fairly uniform throughout the world, affecting 1 in 100 000 of the adult population each year; about 500 new cases of CML are reported annually in the UK. About 2500 new cases of chronic lymphocytic leukaemia (CLL) are diagnosed each year in the UK, but the figures for people in Asia or Africa are much lower. All forms of leukaemia are slightly more common among men than among women.

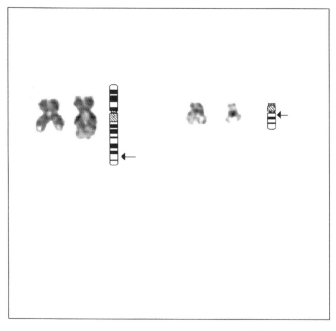

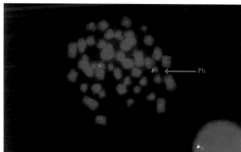

Figure 2.3 The Philadelphia (Ph) chromosome.

What causes leukaemia?

At present no obvious causes of leukaemia have been identified, although several possible causes have been suggested for certain other types of cancers. Many studies of causality have been performed and some of the important ones will be discussed below. However, the most important point to be made here is that, contrary to popular myth, leukaemia, or any other cancer for that matter, is not a punishment for something a patient might have done. Thus patients should not feel guilty about having acquired leukaemia or cancer.

As discussed in the earlier chapter, all cancers, including leukaemias, appear to arise as a consequence of gene mutations. It is likely that the causes of the first mutations are different from subsequent mechanisms which lead to later mutations. The causes are most likely multifactorial. As the world becomes more and more industrialised one can anticipate the number of possible risk factors associated with cancers to increase. It is not uncommon for patients and their relatives to wonder if their life style, particularly their dietary habits and exposure to various chemicals in the environment or at work, may have resulted in their cancers. The various causal pathways of leukaemia are shown diagrammatically in Fig. 2.4.

Agents which result in a cancerous growth are referred to as 'carcinogens' and they seem to result in cancer by two well described pathways. They can damage genes themselves, resulting in mutations, or they can somehow potentiate the growth of the malignant cell.

Based on the diverse molecular abnormalities underlying the cancerous process, it is fairly clear that the majority of gene mutations are acquired after birth and not inherited from parents. There is, of course, a small but significant proportion of cancers which are associated with inherited predisposing

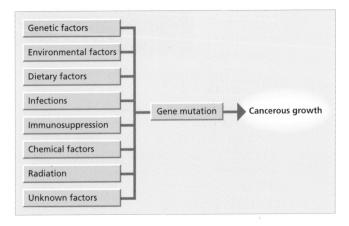

Figure 2.4 Causal pathways resulting in cancer.

genetic conditions. Amongst the leukaemias, it has been established that perhaps up to 5% may arise from inherited abnormal genes. These will be discussed later in this chapter ('Risks from genetic factors').

Risk from radiation

It has long been suspected that radiation may play a role in causing leukaemia. Radiologists and others who were exposed to high levels of irradiation over long periods (before the possible risks were recognised) developed leukaemia more often than would have been expected by chance. Such occupational danger of exposure to ionising radiation is exemplified by the fact that both Marie Curie, who discovered radium one hundred years ago, and her daughter, Irene, both died of leukaemia. Studies in the 1950s by Alice Stewart at Oxford, UK, showed that babies born to women who had diagnostic X-rays in pregnancy (pelvimetry was fashionable then and involved quite high radiation exposures) had an increased risk of acquiring leukaemia five or more years later. Richard Doll recently concluded in his study of *100 Years of Observations on Man of the Hazards of Ionizing Radiation* that the risks of acquiring leukaemia from diagnostic X-rays in pregnancy is increased as the number of exposures increases.

The most compelling link between radiation exposure and leukaemia comes from a Life Span study of the survivors of the atomic bomb explosions in Hiroshima and Nagasaki in 1945. It showed that there is an increased risk of both AML and CML amongst the survivors. It is of interest that investigators did not observe an increased incidence of other cancers, lending weight to the speculation that there are cancer-specific mutations within the target cells (stem cells).

Recently, following the release into the atmosphere of relatively large quantities of radiation, particularly after the explosion at Chernobyl, public interest in the issue of radiation as a cause of leukaemia has been renewed. Studies after the atomic bomb explosions in Japan suggest that a small number of new cases of leukaemia directly attributable to the Chernobyl accident will be seen within the next few years. The early deaths from high exposures to Chernobyl radiation were due to bone marrow failure.

An increased risk of leukaemia has been reported in the area immediately surrounding the British nuclear fuel facility at Calder Hall in Cumbria. Although a government commission of enquiry was unable to confirm a definite increase in the number of cases of leukaemia in the district, the situation nevertheless attracted considerable public attention. Recently a French study linked a possible increase in the incidence of leukaemia among young people in the La Hague area to radioactivity from a reprocessing nuclear plant. Following this report the French government set up a special committee to investigate its findings.

Another area of considerable public concern is the possible role of low energy electromagnetic radiation. The evidence for a possible link with leukaemia is weak, but the results of current case-control studies are eagerly awaited. No link has been established between cosmic ionising radiation (which is greater at high altitude) and leukaemias, although there has been speculation linking radioactive radon gas found in uranium mines and released from granite deposits with the development of leukaemia.

Risks from chemicals

The problems of implicating exposure to toxic chemicals in the development of leukaemia are similar to those concerning radiation. Although there are chemicals that damage the bone marrow and appear to predispose to leukaemia, it is likely that other factors are also important. However, it is impossible to be certain that leukaemia would not have developed in a particular patient in the absence of exposure to the suspect substance.

Aromatic hydrocarbons in general, and benzene and related products in particular, predispose to the development of acute leukaemia. Benzene was formerly used in a number of industrial processes such as in the petroleum industry, in the preparation of photographic film and in the curing of leather. As a result, many workers were exposed to benzene in the first half of this century. A small minority developed blood abnormalities (too few white blood cells or platelets) and even fewer developed acute myeloid leukaemia (AML).

It was noted in laboratory experiments that mouse cells exposed to benzene frequently developed chromosomal abnormalities leading to AML. This provided important circumstantial evidence that this form of AML differed from the usual cases in which there was no exposure to benzene. This supported the suggestion that benzene was at least an important and contributory factor in causing leukaemia. It is now believed that benzene activates an oncogene which causes AML.

Over the past two decades another serious and growing problem has been therapy-induced or 'secondary' leukaemias. Chemicals, such as are used for cytotoxic chemotherapy, and radiotherapy used to treat various cancers may, unfortunately, result in gene mutations which will ultimately result in leukaemias—predominantly AML. The risks involved are generally small, perhaps less than 5%, and the potential benefits from the therapy substantially outweigh this risk. This is a problem particularly when high doses of cytotoxic drugs are used, especially in children being treated for acute lymphoblastic leukaemia (ALL), Hodgkin's disease or other lymphomas. It also appears that radiotherapy may increase the risk of chemotherapy resulting in secondary leukaemias. The latent periods for such leukaemias are quite variable, varying from a year to over 20 years.

More recently another variety of secondary leukaemia with a short latency, usually around 2 years, has been described with two families of drugs called epipodophyllotoxins and anthracyclines. Both of these work against cancer cells by binding to a unique enzyme called topoisomerase II. It has been established that inhibiting this enzyme may trigger DNA breaks and prevent apoptosis, both of which may increase the risk of a secondary cancer developing. Needless to say there is active research going on in this area to improve the benefits of such cancer drugs and to reduce the potential risks. It is possible that some individuals may have an inherited susceptibility which may increase their risk of developing secondary cancers when their first cancers are treated.

Risks from infections

Viruses are fragments of either DNA or ribonucleic acid (RNA) which is another large molecule which acts as a messenger within the cell. Viruses enter cells quite easily and can move from one cell to another and also from person to person.

The compelling idea that viruses may play some part in causing leukaemia was conceived towards the turn of this century. Although viruses are a comparatively recent discovery, it has been known since the end of the last century that undefined infectious organisms could pass through porcelain filters which did not allow bacteria to pass. Initially, the concept that viruses could cause leukaemia or other forms of cancer was widely discounted. Although scientists began to accept that viruses could, under isolated or experimental conditions, cause tumours in animals, they remained sceptical of the association in man. In 1911, Peyton Rous at the Rockefeller Institute in New York had transmitted a cancerous tumour from diseased to normal chickens for the first time. It is interesting to note that Rous received the Nobel Prize for this work 55 years later!

It is still unclear whether any particular virus should be an essential contributory factor in the usual type of sporadic (i.e. primary) leukaemia in man. In the last 20 years, however, it has been established that in the development of at least two rare types of blood cancer described below, viruses (a DNA-containing virus in one and an RNA-containing virus in the other) do indeed play central roles. To understand these two viral-associated lymphoid cancers, it is useful to know that the lymphatic system has several functions, including clearing fluid from around the cells and fighting infection. In a child with tonsillitis, for example, the lymph nodes under the jaw swell in response to the infected material in the tonsils.

Burkitt's lymphoma

In 1957, Denis Burkitt, a British surgeon then working in Uganda, noted that African children between the ages of 3 and 8 years were particularly prone to develop a specific type of tumour involving mainly the bones of the face and the abdominal organs. The common feature of these tumours was that the component cells all seemed to be derived from the lymphatic system. The disease was eventually designated Burkitt's lymphoma. Burkitt was also responsible for appreciating the importance of fibre in our diet—a good example of the value of astute observation of different peoples and cultures.

In 1964, Tony Epstein isolated a DNA-containing virus from tissue cultured from a Ugandan patient with Burkitt's lymphoma. Following additional work by Epstein and his colleague Mollie Barr, this virus was later named the Epstein–Barr virus. Epstein–Barr virus (EBV) has subsequently been found in almost every patient with Burkitt's lymphoma diagnosed in Africa and proteins encoded by the virus are found in the lymphoma cell membranes. The immune systems of these patients also show that they have responded to EBV. It is very likely that EBV is one of the necessary factors contributing to the development of this form of lymphoma in Africa.

Although EBV is widely distributed throughout the world, it usually causes only minor infections in children, and glandular fever (infectious mononucleosis) in adolescents and young adults. Why EBV should cause a relatively benign illness in most individuals but a rare malignant tumour in African children remains unexplained.

Adult T-cell leukaemia/lymphoma
In the late 1970s, doctors in Japan noticed an unusual form of lymphoma. Unlike most lymphatic tumours, which are made up of B-lymphocytes, the unusual Japanese lymphomas were composed of T-lymphocytes. By 1980, Japanese scientists had identified an RNA-containing virus that was present in cells derived from most cases of this newly recognised T-cell lymphoma. The virus was named adult T-cell leukaemia/lymphoma virus (ATLV). An important attribute of ATLV was that it could induce cells to produce an enzyme capable of constructing new sequences of DNA from an RNA model or template. DNA normally directs cells to produce (or transcribe) RNA; there is usually no flow of information from RNA to DNA. For this reason, the enzyme that directs the synthesis of DNA from RNA is known as reverse transcriptase.

Soon after Japanese scientists reported the existence of a virus that was related to this human cancer, a similar virus was isolated from a patient with T-cell leukaemia/lymphoma in the USA. This virus was termed the human T-cell lymphotropic virus (HTLV) and it soon became apparent that

ATLV and HTLV were identical. The virus could be shown to infect normal T-lymphocytes in the test tube, thereby substantially altering their growth characteristics.

Just as EBV causes a particular B-cell cancer in only a few infected people, HTLV causes a specific type of T-cell tumour only in susceptible people. The number of people with antibodies to the virus (evidence that they had been infected in the past) was much larger than the number of those who developed the lymphoma. Clearly, there is more to this than simple infection by these viruses.

The story of HTLV continues to be of great interest. The virus that causes the acquired immune deficiency syndrome (AIDS) was isolated almost simultaneously by Luc Montagnier in Paris and Robert Gallo in the USA. Montagnier called his isolate 'lymphadenopathy-associated virus' or LAV. Gallo noted similarities between the AIDS-related virus and the RNA virus associated with T-cell lymphomas, so he called the T-lymphoma virus HTLV-I and the AIDS-related virus HTLV-III. It now seems that the similarities are not as great as Gallo believed and the AIDS virus has come to be known as the 'human immunodeficiency' virus or HIV—not 'HIV virus' as commonly referred to by the media!

Currently several strains of HTLV have been identified and at least three of these have been causally associated with a variety of cancers arising from the lymphatic system: the HTLV-I has been associated with adult T-cell leukaemia/lymphoma, as described above; the HTLV-II has been implicated in a few cases of prolymphocytic leukaemia and chronic lymphocytic leukaemia, but this finding needs confirmation. Recently researchers from Italy reported a possible link between HTLV-V and a unique lymphoma which affects the skin, cutaneous T-cell lymphoma.

Many specialists believe that the role of infections, particularly those caused by viruses, may be underestimated, especially with regards to the risks of developing lymphoid leukaemias. It is possible that these leukaemias may arise as a consequence of the abnormal immune response. There are a number of interesting epidemiological studies which appear to shed some light on this concept, but direct biological evidence has yet to be established. Researchers are attempting to explain the various 'mini clusters', such as the Sellafield example, by postulating population mixing and viral infections. Currently there are two large studies in progress: a USA based study of some 2500 children with acute leukaemia and a more recent UK study, both seeking to establish the infectious hypothesis as well as population mixing phenomena and other possible risk factors.

Risk of genetic factors

Specialists usually refer to genetic factors as factors that we are born with—those that involve our genes and chromosomes. Recent laboratory research has revealed important clues which implicate genetic factors, in particular those involving gene encoding functions relating to the genes' stability and DNA repair, in the causes of certain kinds of leukaemia. Some individuals who possess either too many or too few chromosomes, or whose chromosomes are weak and disintegrate easily, are at additional risk of acute leukaemia. For example, children born with Down's syndrome, whose genetic make-up is abnormal, are prone to develop acute leukaemia. Children with Fanconi's anaemia have inherited genes resulting in genomic instability and poor DNA repair leading to an extraordinarily high incidence of acute leukaemias (both myeloid and lymphoid).

Interestingly, only very rarely does the identical twin brother or sister of a person with leukaemia also develop leukaemia. This is particularly significant since the only individuals who have exactly the same genes are identical twins. Overall, for the vast majority of patients genetic factors do not appear to play a role in the acquisition of leukaemia. Thus, it is clear that parents of leukaemic children have not bequeathed genetic susceptibility to their offspring.

Risks from dietary factors

Unlike the case in certain common cancers, such as cancers of the lung, throat and bowel, currently there is no known food which increases the risk of acquiring leukaemia. Smoking cigarettes, however, has been implicated in having a causative role in CML. This weak link is dependent on the duration of exposure and, perhaps, the age of starting to smoke.

Despite the lack of an obvious correlation between diet and leukaemias, one should emphasise the paramount importance of a balanced, healthy diet which enables the body's defence systems to operate in a timely and appropriate manner.

3 The different types of leukaemia

Leukaemia can be described as a cancerous change in the early cells from which mature blood cells develop, as discussed in Chapter 1 and shown schematically in Fig. 1.7. The precursor cell from which all blood cells derive is called an haematopoietic stem cell. Stem cells are usually found in the bone marrow and have the ability to develop into either lymphoid precursors, which would normally develop into lymphocytes, or myeloid precursors which would normally become myeloid cells such as granulocytes or monocytes. It is rare for leukaemia to arise simultaneously from both lymphoid and myeloid precursors. Rarely the malignant change occurs in the haematopoietic stem cell, prior to its commitment to either the lymphoid or myeloid lineage.

The marrow of a patient with leukaemia is packed with primitive blast cells (derived from the Greek βλαστανειν 'to grow'), which may also appear in the blood in varying numbers. The effect of this multiplication of leukaemic cells is to interfere with the production of normal blood cells and the patient may therefore become short of red blood cells, white blood cells or platelets, with the effects described in the last chapter.

Leukaemias are generally divided into acute leukaemias and chronic leukaemias. Acute leukaemias are of short duration or rapid onset, whereas chronic leukaemias gradually evolve and are of long duration. Neither term refers to the severity of the disease.

Historically it appears that most of the initial cases of leukaemia described by Virchow, in 1845 were chronic leukaemias. Friedreich appears to have collated the first series of acute leukaemias, in 1857. Most of these appear to have been acute lymphoblastic leukaemia. Myeloblasts were not characterised until 1900, when Naegeli described them. The modern day classification of acute leukaemias, shown in Table 3.1 [known as the French–American–British (FAB) classification, after the

Table 3.1 Classification of ALL by the French–American–British (FAB) criteria

FAB type	Features
L1	Small lymphoblasts; common in children
L2	Medium size blasts; usual adult variety
L3	Burkitt leukaemia; associated with a chromosomal abnormality involving chromosomes number 8 and 14

nationalities of the describing haematologists], did not evolve until 1976.

Acute lymphoblastic leukaemia (ALL)

Acute lymphoblastic leukaemia (ALL) most commonly affects children, particularly those between 2 and 10 years of age. It accounts for 80% of all childhood leukaemias and is the most common type of cancer in children. It also affects adults, mainly those between 30 and 50 years of age, accounting for 20% of all adult leukaemias. The disease is characterised by abnormalities of the lymphoid cell precursors leading to an excessive accumulation of leukaemic lymphoblasts in the marrow and other organs, in particular the spleen and liver.

The annual world-wide incidence of ALL among children is probably about 2.0 per 100 000 persons and about 0.7 per 100 000 adults. The peak incidence in the UK and USA appears to be between the ages of 3 and 5 years. It is of interest to note that in some less affluent countries, such as Turkey, ALL might be less prevalent than acute myeloid leukaemia (AML) in children. The disease seems to afflict more males than females and there appears to be a higher prevalence in Caucasians. ALL has been linked more often than AML to a possible infectious aetiology, in particular viral (EBV) and malaria; in Chapter 2 we also discussed the possible relationship of HTLV-1 to adult ALL.

ALL is divided into a number of different subtypes based upon the clinical and laboratory features. Morphological, molecular and immunological features are particularly important. Most patients can then be classified into various risk groups (prognosis) and the treatment plan is devised accord-

Table 3.2 High risk criteria for patients with ALL

Feature	High risk category	Relative risk
Age	< 2 or > 10 years	1.8
White blood cell count	> 25 × 10^9 per litre	1.9
Chromosomal translocation	Present	2.2
Race	Black	2.5
Organ involvement	CNS 4.0	

CNS, Central Nervous System.

ingly. This is prudent as it enables the individuals with the highest risks to receive the most intensive treatment and vice versa. Table 3.2 summarises the high risk criteria and the 'FAB' classification and Fig. 3.1 shows the morphological appearance of an ALL-L3 subtype. The prognostic features are discussed in detail in Chapter 6 which deals with treatment.

Before effective treatment became available, ALL led to death within weeks of diagnosis, hence it was defined as acute. However, with modern therapy most children can be cured and 'acute' is therefore a less appropriate description than it used to be.

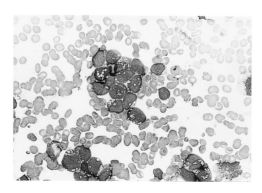

Figure 3.1 A peripheral blood film from a patient with ALL-L3. Note the large leukaemic blast cells with deep blue cytoplasm containing vacuoles and with prominent nuclei.

Acute myeloid leukaemia (AML)

AML, also referred to as acute myelogenous or acute myelocytic leukaemia, is the most common form of acute leukaemia in adults, accounting for over 80% of all acute leukaemias;

Table 3.3 The French–American–British (FAB) classification of AML

FAB type	Features
M1	Undifferentiated—marrow cells show minimal granulocytic maturation
M2	Shows some differentiation; often with an abnormality of chromosomes number 8 and 21
M3	Abnormal promyelocytes with many cytoplasmic granules; often with an abnormality of chromosomes number 15 and 17. Occasionally cells with a different morphology are seen—microgranular with a folded nucleus—this is referred to as M3 variant subtype
M4	Myelo-monocytic; occasionally with increased eosinophils—and an abnormal chromosome number 16 (inverted)—this variety is called M4 Eo
M5	Involves monocytes; often skin and many other organs are infiltrated
M6	Involves red blood cells precursors
M7	Involves platelet precursors (megakaryocytes); bone marrow shows fibrosis

as discussed above, it is encountered less often in children. The overall annual incidence of AML in the UK and USA is about 2.3 per 100 000 persons and it appears to increase with increasing age.

An experienced specialist can, in most cases, easily distinguish the blast cells of AML from those of ALL under the microscope. The distinction is important because different treatments are required. Like ALL, AML was designated as 'acute' at a time when nothing could be done to alter its rapid progression. Today, most AML patients achieve complete remission and become temporarily free of the disease, and some are cured completely.

AML, like ALL, has several subtypes and is classified according to the 'FAB' system, as shown in Table 3.3. In addition there are certain clinical situations that are associated with specific cytogenetic and morphological appearances which deserve special attention as the therapy is often specific and at variance from the other subtypes. For example, AML subtype M3 is characterised by a unique morphology (Fig. 3.2)

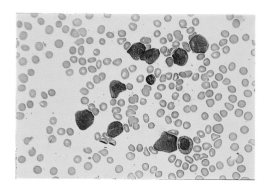

Figure 3.2 A peripheral blood film from a patient with AML-M3. Note the large leukaemic blast cells with pale blue cytoplasm containing many granules. (Courtesy of Dr James Chang, Christie Hospital, Manchester, UK.)

and a translocation involving chromosomes number 15 and 17. The chromosomal breakpoint involves a gene referred to as retinoic acid receptor gene. In 1985, scientists from China observed the favourable response to high doses of a specific type of retinoic acid termed all-*trans*-retinoic acid (ATRA, a derivative of vitamin A) in patients demonstrating these abnormalities.

Recent molecular genetic studies of different cases of AML have revealed that several chromosomal translocations involve the same breakpoint, implicating this as a potential AML gene. The identity of this gene has now been established as acute myeloid leukaemia 1 (AML-1). It is located on chromosome number 21 and is found in 20% of AML patients, particularly those with AML M2. These (latter) patients have a translocation involving chromosomes number 8 and 21. Curiously the presence of this chromosome abnormality usually confers a relatively good prognosis on these patients.

Hybrid leukaemia

Rarely there appears to be a simultaneous presence of both lymphoid and myeloid leukaemic cells. The leukaemia is then referred to as 'biclonal' (two clones). In rare instances the leukaemia arises from one precursor, but the blast cells express both lymphoid and myeloid markers. This is called hybrid (or biphenotypic) leukaemia. The significance of these unique situations is not clear and in general, therapy is tailored according to the dominant features.

Chronic lymphocytic leukaemia (CLL)

Chronic lymphocytic leukaemia (CLL) or, as it used to be called, chronic lymphatic leukaemia, is the most common type of leukaemia in the western world and mainly affects people over the age of 40. In the US, about 10 000 new cases are diagnosed each year. Unlike the other leukaemias, CLL is not induced by exposure to any known chemicals or radiation. Recently there was speculation that CLL might be causally linked to infection by HTLV-I, based upon a small Jamaican study, but this remains unconfirmed.

CLL is characterised by an increased number of normal-looking but biologically immature B-lymphocytes in the blood and bone marrow (Fig. 3.3). Since CLL is a disease of the B-lymphocytes, it is not surprising to see a host of immunological problems in patients with CLL. These may result in frequent bacterial infections and other auto-immune disorders whereby individuals make antibodies which attack their own organs. Recently a number of chromosomal abnormalities, for example trisomy 12 (an 'extra' chromosome number 12), have been described in CLL (see Fig. 3.4).

CLL is usually a relatively mild disease and some patients survive for many years with minimal or no treatment. In other cases, however, the disease is more aggressive and frequent treatment is required. Either way, the patient may survive a number of years after diagnosis and hence the disease is considered chronic. Due to these variable presentations, it is important to group patients according to their risk factors and

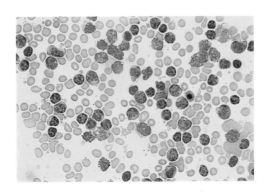

Figure 3.3 A peripheral blood film from a patient with CLL.

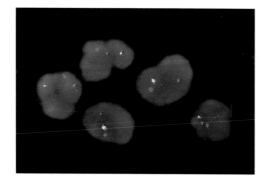

Figure 3.4 Chromosomal abnormality—trisomy 12—in a patient with CLL.

then to individualise therapy. This is often done using a staging system called Rai's classification (see Table 3.4). Rarely CLL can transform into other types of lymphoid malignancies, usually non-Hodgkin's lymphoma; there have even been reports of CLL transforming to ALL. Figure 3.5 shows massive enlargement of neck lymph nodes in a patient with CLL which has transformed into a non-Hodgkin's lymphoma.

There are two other kinds of chronic leukaemias related to CLL: prolymphocytic leukaemia and hairy cell leukaemia. Prolymphocytic leukaemia (PLL) was first described by Galton at the Hammersmith Hospital in London in 1974. He and his colleagues observed that some patients who were initially

35

Table 3.4 Rai's staging system for CLL

Stage	Criteria	Average survival (years)
0 (low risk)	Lymphocytes > 15 × 20^9/l Bone marrow > 40% lymphocyte	> 10
I & II (intermediate risk)	As stage 0 plus lymph node enlargement & liver or spleen enlargement	6
III & IV (high risk)	As stage I & II plus haemoglobin < 11 g/dl or platelets < 100 × 10^9/l	2

thought to have CLL had a number of characteristics not seen in patients with CLL. The lymphocyte counts almost always number more than 100×10^9/l and consist of cells which appear more immature and are larger than CLL cells (see Fig. 3.6, which shows a peripheral blood film from a patient with PLL). These patients often have greater spleen and liver enlargement and, interestingly, lymph node enlargement is either minimal or absent. Most patients with PLL tend to be over

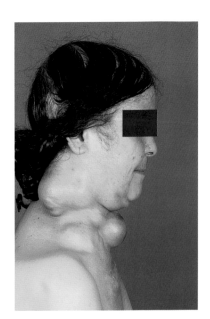

Figure 3.5 Massive enlargement of neck lymph nodes in a patient with CLL which has transformed into a non-Hodgkin's lymphoma.

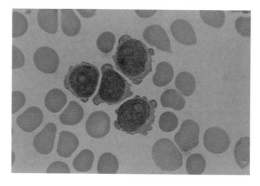

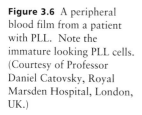

Figure 3.6 A peripheral blood film from a patient with PLL. Note the immature looking PLL cells. (Courtesy of Professor Daniel Catovsky, Royal Marsden Hospital, London, UK.)

the age of 60 years. There are two distinct subtypes of PLL: B-cell and T-cell types. The T-cell type has been causally associated with infection with HTLV-II. Many patients have a chromosomal abnormality involving chromosome number 14 (14q+).

Hairy cell leukaemia was described by Bouroncle and her colleagues in 1958. It is an exceedingly rare disease accounting for about 1% of all leukaemias, but has fascinated many researchers and clinicians by virtue of its several unique features. Most patients tend to be aged between 50 and 70 years and males are more often affected than females. The typical hairy leukaemia cell is an irregular cell with a serrated or 'tentacled' border (see Fig. 3.7, which shows a peripheral blood film from a patient with hairy cell leukaemia). The cytoplasm of the cell is sky blue and devoid of any granules. When these cells are examined under an electron microscope, long cytoplasmic villi resembling tentacles or hairs are seen (hence the name—hairy cell). Figure 3.8 shows the peripheral blood of a patient with hairy cell leukaemia seen by electron microscopy. Most patients present with weakness and fatigue. Clinically most have an enlarged spleen, which is often huge, and normally there is no lymph node enlargement.

Another rare form of chronic leukaemia related to CLL is the adult T-cell leukaemia/lymphoma (ATL) which was described in the previous chapter (pages 25–26). This disease is associated with infection by HTLV-I. Although first described in patients from the Caribbean and Japan, it has since been reported world-wide. The average age of the patients is around 40 years and men appear to be at higher risk than women.

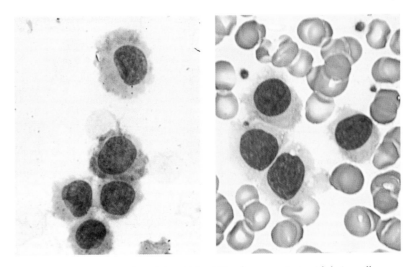

Figure 3.7 A peripheral blood film from a patient with hairy cell leukaemia. Note the cells with a serrated border and a sky-blue cytoplasm without granules.

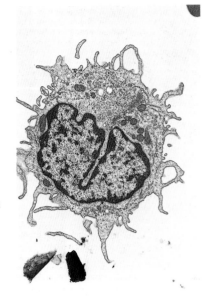

Figure 3.8 A peripheral blood film from a patient with hairy cell leukaemia seen by electron microscopy, magnified 17 000 times. Note the hair-like pseudopods projecting out of the cell surface. (Courtesy of Professor Daniel Catovsky, Royal Marsden Hospital, London, UK.)

38

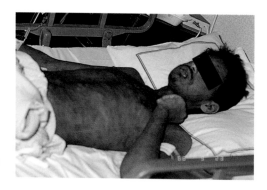

Figure 3.9 Skin involvement in a patient with ATL.

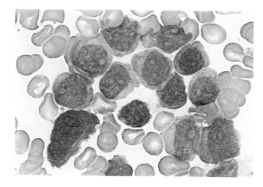

Figure 3.10 A peripheral blood film from a patient with ATL. Note the multi-lobular nuclei. (Courtesy of Professor Daniel Catovsky, Royal Marsden Hospital, London, UK.)

Most patients present with lymph node enlargement and high lymphocyte counts. About two-thirds of patients have a peculiar skin involvement (see Fig. 3.9) which can sometimes be confused with cutaneous T-cell lymphoma. Another important feature of ATL is the presence of characteristic abnormal circulating lymphocytes. Figure 3.10 shows the peripheral blood film from a typical patient showing ATL cells with multilobular nuclei. Patients with ATL can sometimes present with high blood calcium levels which can result in weakness, lethargy and even confusion.

Chronic myeloid leukaemia (CML)

Chronic myeloid leukaemia (CML) accounts for about 15% of all cases of leukaemia in the West and probably 25% of cases in the Orient. It has an annual world-wide incidence of about 1 per 100 000 persons and is especially prevalent in young adults, but is rare in children. There is a small but significant increased risk of developing CML following excessive exposure to radiation, as in the Hiroshima and Nagasaki experience (see Chapter 2).

CML is probably one of the best understood human cancers. Although first described as a discrete entity in 1845, significant progress in understanding CML did not occur until 1960 with the discovery of the Philadelphia chromosome in patients with CML (see Fig. 2.3). In 1973, it was shown that the Philadelphia chromosome was due to a reciprocal translocation involving chromosomes number 9 and 22. Thereafter it was established that this translocation was causally linked with CML. The past two decades have witnessed the unravelling of the molecular mechanisms underlying CML. Two specific genes, the ABL gene normally present on chromosome number 9 and the BCR gene normally present on chromosome number 22, are involved in this translocation. Both genes are transected in the formation of the translocation and parts of both genes are linked in sequence (juxtaposed) on the Philadelphia chromosome. This results in new BCR-ABL fusion gene that produces a specific protein (called P210). The P210 probably plays a major role in the process that leads to CML. Interestingly, a similar but slightly smaller protein, termed P190, has been found in 60–70% of the cases of patients with ALL who have a Philadelphia chromosome. Recently, a slightly larger related protein, termed P230, was found in patients with a very rare indolent leukaemia called chronic neutrophilic leukaemia.

In CML the bone marrow is almost entirely replaced by myeloid cells of the granulocyte lineage. The megakaryocytes (parent cells of platelets) are increased in number and the white blood cells are usually increased to between 10 and 25 times normal. The spleen is also enlarged, often substantially. Nevertheless, as many as 40% of patients have no symptoms when first seen and the diagnosis is made following the observation of a high white cell count (leucocytosis) in a routine blood test.

Because untreated patients may survive for some years, CML was once considered chronic and the label has stuck. It was believed, incorrectly, that due to its slow natural evolution, this form of leukaemia was less aggressive. Further confusion has arisen over the past decade with the vast improvements seen in the treatment of some acute leukaemias. Because of these advances the survival rates in many patients with acute leukaemia are better than those for CML patients. In fact, until a decade ago, CML was generally regarded as incurable; today, an appreciable number of patients who have had a bone marrow transplant can be considered cured.

CML is characterised by two, or sometimes three, fairly distinct phases: an initial insidious or chronic phase with an average duration of 4–5 years, usually followed by an abrupt transition to an aggressive form. This transition is termed the 'blast crisis' and results in a particularly severe form of CML, which leads to death in most patients within a matter of months. Sometimes the insidious phase is followed by a gradual transition to blast crisis. This may take many months and is termed the 'accelerated phase'.

4 Diagnosis of leukaemia

Initial symptoms

The way in which leukaemia first shows itself varies and depends to a considerable extent on the type of disease. Patients with acute leukaemia may have one or more symptoms that develop suddenly and require urgent medical attention, whereas those with one of the chronic leukaemias are more likely to gradually feel increasingly tired or poorly. Indeed, they may have no symptoms at all when their disease is diagnosed following a routine blood examination. **It is important to remember that most patients with these nonspecific symptoms do not have leukaemia and that leukaemias are not common conditions.**

One of the most common initial features in children with ALL is anaemia. Anaemic people may look pale, may become easily tired and, in some cases, may be short of breath. Alternatively, they may have unprovoked or inappropriate bleeding from unusual places such as their gums, intestine or skin, or they may become unduly susceptible to infections, developing abscesses or pneumonia, or a fever without an obvious cause. Sometimes pains in the arms and legs mimic arthritis or bone infection, in which case leukaemia may not be suspected. Table 4.1 shows the most common presenting symptoms in children with ALL.

Table 4.1 Presenting symptoms of children with ALL

Symptom	Frequency (%)
Fever	60
Tiredness	60
Bleeding	40
Bone pain	30
Joint pain	20
Anorexia	20
Abdominal pain	10

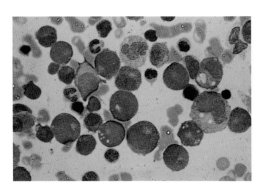

Figure 4.1 A peripheral blood film from a patient with AML-M2. Note the large blast cells with folded nuclei and granules in the cytoplasm.

Adults with AML may consult their doctors with any of the same nonspecific symptoms that affect children with ALL. However, bone and joint pains are much less common in AML than in ALL, whereas bleeding problems are more common. Most patients give a short history of such symptoms, usually of a few weeks to a few months. AML rarely presents as an incidental finding on a routine blood test. Patients with AML subtype M3 usually present with extensive bleeding and sometimes with inappropriate thrombosis (clotting). This is due to unique granules within the leukaemic cells (see Fig. 3.2), which trigger bleeding and thrombosis (paradoxically) on being released into the bloodstream. Over a third of all AML patients have a serious infection, usually bacterial, at the time of presentation. The most common sites of such infections are chest, bladder, skin and sinuses. The mouth is often involved with a fungal infection (candida or thrush). Figure 4.1 shows the typical peripheral blood findings from a patient afflicted with AML-M2.

Often, particularly in the AML subtypes M4 and M5, leukaemic cells infiltrate the skin (referred to as leukaemia cutis, see Fig. 4.2), gums (gingival hypertrophy; see Fig. 4.3) and tonsils. When leukaemic cells involve adenoids and tonsils, they can cause serious airway obstruction. The spleen is enlarged in 25% of patients with AML.

Occasionally, in both ALL and in AML, and especially in subtypes M4 and M5, patients present with central nervous system (CNS) involvement by the leukaemic cells. This usually results from infiltration of the meninges or lining of the

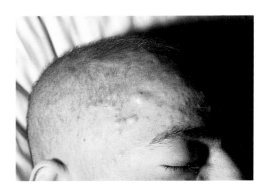

Figure 4.2 A photograph showing leukaemia cutis in a patient with AML. Note how prominent the skin nodules are.

brain, and contamination of the fluid which circulates around the brain and spinal cord (the cerebrospinal fluid or CSF). Rarely the CNS involvement is actually due to the very large number of leukaemic cells within the brain circulation causing the blood flow to be sluggish; this is referred to as leucostasis.

Both ALL and AML can also involve other organs. For example testicular leukaemic infiltration has been observed in young boys. This is far more common in ALL but can be seen with AML M4 and M5. Other organ involvement is less common.

Patients with CML may become tired so gradually, over a period of 3–12 months, that they hardly notice the deterioration in their health. They may eventually become short of breath, lose weight or sweat excessively. If the spleen becomes large enough, patients will notice it as a swelling in their

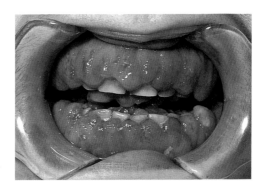

Figure 4.3 A photograph showing gum hypertrophy in a patient with AML-M5.

abdomen. As in patients with acute leukaemia, another first symptom in patients with CML is inappropriate bleeding.

Because of the slow onset of the disease, CML may be diagnosed from a blood test performed for another purpose, such as before surgery, in the ante-natal clinic or during routine medical examination. About 1% of males present with priapism, which is a painful erect penis that does not subside. This rare and embarrassing problem is usually preceded by a short history, of days to a few weeks, of less troublesome intermittent but prolonged penile erections. Over 80% of CML patients will have some splenic enlargement and in about 20% the spleen is greatly enlarged and may occupy over half of the abdominal cavity.

Patients with CLL are most likely to be diagnosed as a result of a chance blood test, although they may develop general symptoms such as loss of appetite, loss of weight or undue sweating, especially at night. Alternatively, localised symptoms such as enlarged lymph nodes in the side of the neck, under the arms or in the groin, or an enlarged spleen may alert them to the problem. Some patients with CLL have increased susceptibility to infections, especially bacterial, and will often present with chest or bladder infections. In due course, as the disease progresses, most patients develop infections.

Laboratory tests

The diagnosis of leukaemia is usually made by examination of blood taken from a vein in the arm. The number of white blood cells in the blood normally ranges from 4000 to 10 000 per cubic millimetre. Patients with leukaemia frequently have increased white blood cell counts, usually in the range of 20 000–200 000 per cubic millimetre. This is the finding that usually attracts the specialist's attention. There are many other causes for a moderately raised white blood cell count (up to about 20 000 per cubic millimetre) but very high levels are most likely to be due to leukaemia.

The next step is to examine the blood under a microscope. Although special stains are used to enable the various types of cell to be identified, it is not always possible to tell which type

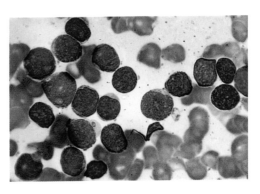

Figure 4.4 Peripheral blood findings from a patient with acute undifferentiated leukaemia. (Courtesy of Professor Daniel Catovsky, Royal Marsden Hospital, London, UK.)

of white blood cell predominates. However, if most of the white blood cells are of the immature variety (blast cells), then the diagnosis of acute leukaemia is almost certain. Figure 4.4 shows blast cells from a patient suffering from acute undifferentiated leukaemia. In most cases the blast cells are differentiated and it is possible to differentiate AML from ALL by examining the patient's blood, although occasionally the distinction is difficult and further tests are required. If the white blood cell count is over 50 000 per cubic millimetre, the diagnosis of CML (see Fig. 4.5) or CLL is usually straightforward.

Occasionally, the leucocyte count is normal in a patient who has other blood abnormalities that might indicate the presence of leukaemia. In such cases, examination of the bone marrow is necessary to confirm (or exclude) the diagnosis. In practice, examination of the marrow is carried out routinely in all newly diagnosed patients, even when the diagnosis has

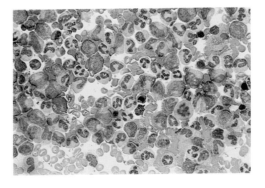

Figure 4.5 A peripheral blood film from a patient with CML. Note that cells of all stages in granulopoietic development are present.

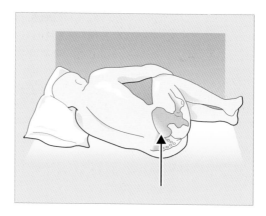

Figure 4.6 How a bone marrow examination is carried out.

already been established by blood examination, because it gives a great deal of extra information that is necessary in planning the treatment.

Marrow examination is relatively simple. The doctor or a Specialist Nurse anaesthetises the skin over the back of the hip bone and inserts a medical needle until it touches the bone (see Fig. 4.6). The needle is then gradually advanced through the thick layer of outer bone and into the spongy cavity that contains the marrow. A syringe attached to the needle is used to suck out about 3–5 ml of marrow cells mixed with blood. These marrow cells are then stained (to bring out detail) and examined under a microscope. The marrow of patients with acute leukaemia is densely packed with cells, most of them blast cells. This is very different from the appearance of normal marrow, in which cells of many different shapes and sizes are seen in different proportions (see Fig. 4.7). Marrow packed

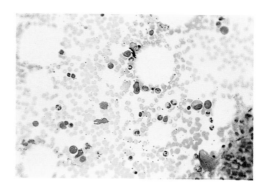

Figure 4.7 A thin section of a normal bone marrow; magnified 50 times. Note that cells of many different shapes and sizes are present.

with leukaemic cells is occasionally found even when no blast cells are found in the patient's blood.

The marrow of patients with chronic leukaemia is similar to that seen in acute leukaemia in that it is densely packed with cells but in CML, the cells are granulocytes in all stages of maturation, similar to those seen in the blood. In CLL, the cells normally present in the marrow are replaced to varying degrees by small lymphocytes similar to those found in excess in the blood. The proportion of lymphocytes in the marrow may range from 40% to 90%.

It is customary to carry out a battery of specialised tests to establish the identity and the presence (or absence) of various immunological markers on the leukaemic cell surface or inside the cell. Nowadays most specialist laboratories use a panel of monoclonal antibodies which enable the haematologist to determine the nature of the leukaemic cells. These reagents are usually employed with flow cytometers, which have considerable advantages over traditional microscopy, particularly the speed of analysis and the accurate quantitative assessment of the cells.

Many other tests are available to help the specialist characterise the leukaemic cells more precisely, to provide information that may be useful in planning the treatment, and for research purposes (any test conducted purely for research does, of course, require the patient's consent). For example, tests can be performed to determine which of a number of possible enzymes are present in the cytoplasm of the leukaemic cells, and whether or not certain 'marker' proteins produced only by abnormal cells are present on the cell surface.

A particularly valuable test is to examine the chromosomal make-up of the leukaemic cells which can be carried out on a specimen of the patient's bone marrow aspirate; it can also be performed using a blood sample, if the leukaemic cell count is high. Figure 3.4 shows a fairly common chromosomal abnormality seen in patients with CLL, trisomy 12, which often confers a poorer prognosis.

An increasing number of specialist laboratories, at least in developed countries, are using DNA-based techniques to help the specialist identify the precise genes afflicted and to characterise the leukaemia accordingly. We can anticipate a greater use of such tests as some of the fruits of our increasing under-standing of leukaemogenesis ultimately translates to some clinical and more importantly, therapeutic relevance. We will discuss these aspects further in Chapter 6.

5 The patient and the doctor

The diagnosis of leukaemia is often made in a roundabout way. Initially a patient may be referred from one (unfamiliar) hospital to another, before he receives any real explanation. The news usually comes as a (psychological) bombshell to both the patient and his or her relatives, and, perhaps, as a total surprise to the family physician. Most patients are deeply upset and may even be resentful. If they feel that the diagnosis was delayed for some time, they may wonder whether their chances of being cured have been jeopardised by the delay. Some patients will be annoyed to see most, if not all, previously performed tests repeated at the specialised centre. Naturally, most patients and their relatives may feel despondent. The patients will wonder why it happened to them; they may feel guilt that the disease is due to something they have done or could have avoided doing. Parents may ask 'Why *my* child?' and wonder if other family members will be affected. The specialist therefore is faced not only with the difficult task of informing the patient and his or her relatives about the diagnosis but also with helping them to cope with the news. The specialist's approach is likely to be guided by the type of leukaemia, as well as by the patient's age, clinical condition, and ability to understand.

If ALL is diagnosed in a child, the specialist will probably talk first with the parents and explain the treatment strategy and prognosis. At this stage, and perhaps also later, the specialist will probably also emphasise that statistics relate only imprecisely to individual patients, and that, while there is a very good chance that the child will be cured, the possibility of failure must not be entirely discounted.

How much a doctor will choose to tell a young patient depends very much on the individual circumstances; however, it may be perfectly reasonable to explain to a child that he or she has a disease that may be fatal if appropriate treatment is not given. This should certainly help to emphasise to the child the need to collaborate in the treatment programme.

Patients with AML are more likely to be adults than children. Even though 20–30 years ago it was customary to conceal the diagnosis from patients and to inform only relatives; today it is normal practice, at least in North America and most parts of Europe, to give the newly diagnosed patient details of the diagnosis and to explain some basic features about the biology of the disease, and the treatment that will be used to try to achieve remission and, hopefully, cure.

The most difficult question of all is when the patient finally asks 'Doctor, how long do I have to live?'. It is always impossible to give an accurate answer to this question and therefore the best approach is for the doctor to explain the expected range of survival, i.e. that one patient may die within a few weeks of diagnosis whereas another may eventually be cured.

A frank discussion at the time of diagnosis is equally important for the patient with CML or CLL, even if he or she had absolutely no symptoms when the diagnosis was made. The doctor will almost certainly draw attention to the fact that chronic means slowly progressive, and will explain the implications of this. The patient with CML will be told about the two, or sometimes three, stage nature of the disease and the unpredictability of the onset of transformation. When talking to a patient with CLL, the doctor should stress that some patients live 20 or more years following diagnosis, though the average survival is less.

Many patients want to know about the causes both of leukaemia in general and of their own disease in particular. Most doctors will explain the possible roles of environmental factors such as radiation, toxic chemicals and viruses, but they will also admit that it is almost always impossible to determine the true contribution of such factors in individual cases.

Most patients are well informed generally and will not expect striking revelations about their disease. However, two aspects about the development of leukaemia may be of particular importance and are worth stressing. First, many patients with children are concerned that there may be a risk that is passed on genetically; however, until we know much more about the causes of leukaemia, we can say quite simply that the risk of it occurring twice in one family is only very slightly greater than one would expect from chance alone.

Secondly, patients may be concerned that a chemical with which they have come into contact may have caused or contributed to their leukaemia. In most cases, the doctor is asked about the possible role of a specific chemical; usually, however, it is difficult for the doctor to give an answer because no clear evidence exists one way or the other. However, if a patient has been exposed to benzene or a closely related compound, he or she may well be entitled to compensation from an employer, and legal advice should be sought. Some people are concerned about whether leukaemia is contagious and they should be reassured that no leukaemia can be caught from, or passed on to, another person.

Finally, specialists recognise that most patients are stunned by the diagnosis and in their bewildered state may only comprehend part of the discussions which take place. Most specialists will be very accommodating and encourage the patients and their relatives to ask questions; moreover, they will understand that much of what is said initially may need to be repeated later. The specialist may also suggest contacting a variety of support organisations, such as the Leukaemia Society in the USA, the Leukaemia Research Fund and the Leukaemia Care Society in the UK and various regional organisations. For the convenience of the reader, some of the support organisations in the UK and USA, with the appropriate means of contact, are listed in Appendix 1. The family unit is probably the most important source of support together with the specialist team. The team should not only be accessible and compassionate but should be prepared to offer referral to other sources of support, such as religious groups.

6 The treatment of leukaemia

Introduction

Treatment is usually given soon after diagnosis for patients with all kinds of acute leukaemias and CML. In CLL, with the exception of the subtype called hairy cell leukaemia, treatment is usually only required in the more advanced stages because there is no evidence that treatment early in the disease is beneficial. The mainstay of all leukaemia treatment is chemotherapy, which simply means the use of drugs to treat a sickness.

The cancer chemotherapy drugs given to patients with acute leukaemias are very different from those used to treat chronic leukaemias, but they have some things in common. They usually work by disrupting the ability of the cancer cells to grow and multiply. They can be given by several routes. When given by mouth, chemotherapeutic agents are absorbed into the bloodstream from the gut and are carried throughout the body to reach the cancer cells. Drugs that cannot be given by mouth, either because they are destroyed in the stomach and gut or because they are not well absorbed, are injected into muscles or veins. In practice, most drugs given to patients with leukaemia are injected or infused directly into a vein; that way they reach cancer cells very rapidly and can begin to work without delay.

All chemotherapy drugs have their own specific modes of action; some kill leukaemic cells only when they are multiplying, while others kill all leukaemic cells. They can be used singly or in groups that work together, i.e. as combination chemotherapy. Most treatment plans for leukaemia include combination chemotherapy and, occasionally, radiation therapy. Such treatment plans are known as combined modality treatments.

The quantity of each drug used in a combination is calculated for each patient according to his or her height and weight.

The amount of a particular drug that can be used also depends on how the body reacts to it. Unfortunately, these drugs do not discriminate accurately between normal and leukaemic cells, so all cells are affected to some degree and considerable damage can occur to normal tissue in which cell division is rapid. Cells that are particularly susceptible are those in the lining of the mouth and gut, the skin, and the bone marrow. Most of the side-effects are unpleasant but are usually reversible and generally not serious. However, very rarely, serious complications do happen, so it is sensible for all patients who require intensive combination therapy to be treated where expert medical help and extensive supportive care are available if required.

Patients with leukaemia often first seek medical help because of an emergency such as life-threatening bleeding or serious infection which have to be dealt with before specific antileukaemic therapy can be given.

It should also be said that although the treatment of leukaemias has improved considerably in the last decade, the overall results are still not entirely satisfactory. It is for this reason that many new treatments are under investigation, and it is desirable for most patients to enter 'clinical trials'. Clinical trials offer potential value to both patients and specialists. They offer the patient variations that may improve on established treatment or, occasionally, a completely new therapy. At the same time, they enable the specialist to evaluate new treatments. Clinical trials are carefully controlled: the patient (or guardian) must agree to entry into the trial by signing an (informed) consent form; the trial itself must first be approved by a supervisory panel which is made up of individuals who are not involved in the trial itself. In most countries, these panels include ethicists and other nonmedical members. There is also a monitoring body, usually a group of specialists in the field who are independent of the trial members, who follow the results and stop the trial if the results of the new regimen prove to be superior to the old (in which case the new regimen will become the standard treatment) or if the results are poorer (in which case the trial will be abandoned). Perhaps it should be mentioned that nearly all advances in the treatment of leukaemia have been made through clinical trials. In the

UK, the largest trials are organised by the Medical Research Council (MRC), and at present 90% of the children diagnosed as having ALL are entered into MRC trials.

The treatment of both acute and chronic leukaemias requires a multidisciplinary approach with a first rate supportive care facility. The treatment in general tends to be long and requires repeated hospital admissions. Moreover, regular medical supervision will be required, quite possibly for life. The outlook is influenced mainly by age and factors related to the biology of the disease.

The goal of therapy in acute leukaemias is to reduce and eradicate the leukaemic cells while preserving the normal cells. A common denominator for the success of all leukaemia therapy is the coexistence of normal and leukaemic cells at diagnosis. It is then anticipated that effective therapy will sufficiently reduce the leukaemic cells to allow the normal cells to grow.

In order to facilitate good vascular access, most patients with acute leukaemia require an indwelling central venous catheter soon after main diagnosis has been confirmed. Catheters, such as the Hickman catheter (see Fig. 6.1), are usually inserted by a Specialist Nurse or a Surgeon, using local or general anaesthetic. These are used for taking blood samples and for giving intravenous fluids, chemotherapy, antibiotics and blood products. The tip of the catheter is usually positioned at the entrance to the right atrium (the smaller right-sided chamber of the heart, through which all the blood returns). In order to offer maximum use, most catheters comprise either double or triple tubes, each for injection of different materials. These catheters can remain in place for periods of 6–9 months, and sometimes even longer, without any complications. They do, however, require careful maintenance, particularly when home care is required. Patients are taught not only to change dressings but also about flushing methods (in order to keep the tubes open). Activities such as bathing, swimming, sexual intercourse, etc. can be enjoyed without any risk of damaging the catheter.

Sometimes specialists may select a catheter which is connected to a small implantable port (such as Port-A-Cath; see Fig. 6.2). This is a device implanted underneath the skin (subcutaneously) and is particularly suitable for patients receiving

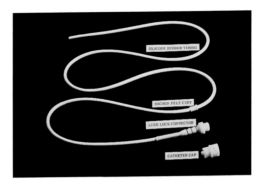

(a)

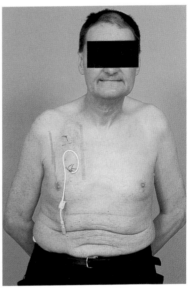

Figure 6.1 *(a) and (b)* A
Hickman catheter.

(b)

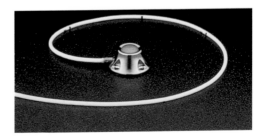

Figure 6.2 A Port-A-Cath.

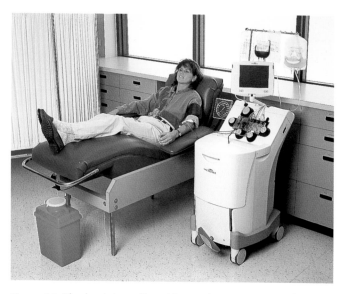

Figure 6.3 Platelets being collected from a donor. (Courtesy of Mr Edward Wood, COBE Laboratories, Lakewood, Colorado, USA.)

less intensive treatment, usually on an outpatient basis. Most implantable ports have a single tube or lumen, but double lumen ports are also available. The main advantage of these devices compared to external catheters, such as the Hickman, are the ease of maintenance and cosmetic appearance.

Most patients with acute leukaemia present with symptoms such as fever, infection and bleeding which often need to be dealt with immediately. They will require the prompt placement of a central venous catheter, as discussed above. Most patients will require transfusions, usually of red blood cells and platelets. Figure 6.3 shows a platelet collection being carried out. Nowadays all blood products are filtered (to reduce the chances of being contaminated by white blood cells which can result in allergic and febrile transfusion reactions) and irradiated in order to destroy any lymphocytes of donor origin which might be present in the transfused blood. These lymphocytes have the potential to mount a harmful reaction against the recipient, called graft-vs-host disease. This will be discussed in the next chapter which deals with bone marrow transplantation. Irradiation of blood products before they are administered to the patient is considered totally safe.

A serious but usually preventable complication can occasionally result from treatment. This is termed the tumour lysis syndrome and it may occur spontaneously or shortly after therapy has begun. The syndrome is due to the rapid destruction (lysis) of leukaemic cells as a result of treatment, resulting in the liberation of vast quantities of cellular material which overwhelms the filtration system in the kidneys. This leads to a number of clinical abnormalities: high levels of potassium, low calcium, high phosphorus and high uric acid and, if left untreated, this syndrome can result in catastrophic consequences. Specialists will therefore take appropriate precautions when treating patients with large tumour burdens (those with very high white cell counts) prior to commencing intensive treatment.

Another potentially difficult problem is the emergence of drug resistance. In much the same way as bacteria develop resistance to antibiotics, leukaemic cells can develop resistance to drugs. The mechanisms involved are usually multiple. It is not unusual for leukaemic cells to become drug resistant by altering their enzymes. For example, methotrexate resistance is associated with alteration of an enzyme (called dihydrofolate reductase) which is essential for the activity of the drug. The leukaemic cell is able to increase the quantity of this enzyme by activating the responsible gene; additionally there is a qualitative alteration of the enzyme. Similarly, resistance can develop to the drug Ara-C by the cell increasing the level of another enzyme (cytidine deaminase) which is essential for the action of this drug, and alterations to another enzyme, topoisomerase II (see page 23) results in resistance to the epipodophyllotoxins (such as etoposide) and anthracyclines (such as daunorubicin).

Another unique mechanism for drug resistance has been discovered recently. It was observed that when cancer cells are exposed to certain cytotoxic drugs they develop resistance to several other, often unrelated, drugs due to alterations to the multidrug resistance (mdr) gene. When the mdr gene is altered, it results in the overproduction of a protein termed P glycoprotein which confers resistance to the cancer cells by enhancing the cellular elimination of cytotoxic drugs. Mdr affects drugs such as the vinca alkaloids, anthracyclines and epipodophyllotoxins. Researchers have developed a number of novel methods to circumvent this type of drug resistance, for example by treating patients with drugs known as calcium-channel blockers, often used by cardiologists to treat heart rhythm disorders (such as verapamil). Several clinical studies exploring other novel ways of combating mdr are in progress.

The treatment of ALL

The treatment of ALL is directed first at trying to destroy all the leukaemic cells in the bone marrow and lymphoid system, and, secondly, at destroying any leukaemia cells that are left in so-called 'sanctuary sites'. These are parts of the body, including the testes, ovaries, brain and spinal cord, where leukaemic cells are found but where it is difficult to achieve high concentrations of antileukaemic drugs. Leukaemic cells can reside in sanctuaries, in a resting state (G_0 phase; see page 16), for prolonged periods prior to beginning to proliferate again and causing a clinical relapse.

The treatment outcome of ALL has improved substantially over the past 3–4 decades, particularly in children in whom the survival has improved from a few weeks to cure in 65–70% of cases. In adults success has been considerably less but both the remission rates and probability of cure do appear to be rising. For patients with high-risk prognostic features there are now a number of different therapeutic strategies.

The conventional approach is a treatment plan in three phases: remission induction, consolidation and maintenance. Induction, which usually involves the use of three or four drugs, commonly results in complete remission, which is defined as the absence of detectable leukaemic cells in the blood and bone marrow. Complete remission is usually achieved in more than 90% of children and 60% of adults who do not have high-risk factors (see Table 3.2). Patients who are at high risk require more intensive treatment.

Once complete remission is achieved, several extra courses of the same drugs are given to minimize likelihood of recurrence of the disease. This is referred to as consolidation. The most commonly used drugs in the first and second phases of treatment are vincristine, daunorubicin (or its equivalent), L-asparaginase, and prednisolone. Prednisolone is given by mouth and the other three drugs by injection into a vein.

Vincristine is a potent cancer chemotherapeutic drug extracted from the periwinkle plant *Vinca rosea*. It works directly on leukaemic cells by binding to the protein tubulin and preventing cellular division. Tubulin forms fibres (as its name implies) that help cell division to progress in an orderly fashion. Since all leukaemic cells do not divide at the same time, vincristine is given weekly in the hope that eventually all the leukaemic cells will be affected. Vincristine can cause constipation and stomach cramps. Given in excess, it can lead to temporary paralysis of the bowel or of certain nerves, resulting in muscle weakness which may result in foot-drop, wrist-drop, and facial paralysis. Most of these effects are completely reversible and are rarely seen in current treatment schedules.

Daunorubicin is an anthracycline that acts directly by inhibiting cell growth by blocking the action of the enzyme topoisomerase II, which was mentioned in Chapter 2. Drugs which inhibit this powerful enzyme prevent repair of broken DNA strands, resulting in cell death. It gives the urine a harmless reddish colour which may persist for 24–48 h. The drug has several common side-effects including nausea, vomiting and bone marrow depression. On rare occasions, it can also damage the heart, particularly if given in large amounts. Specialists are therefore careful not to give too large a dose, or they may use a cardioprotectant (such as Cardioxane, an experimental drug) concomitantly.

Over the past few years a number of new generation anthracyclines have become available such as epirubicin and idarubicin. These agents appear to be less harmful to the heart and idarubicin also appears to be more potent in killing leukaemic cells. An increasing number of specialists now use idarubicin instead of daunorubicin. Another related drug, mitozantrone, may also have fewer toxic effects than daunorubicin. Mitozantrone belongs to another family (anthraquinones) but resembles anthracyclines in chemical structure and function. It has proven to be very useful as a second-line drug for patients with ALL and AML and is being investigated as a possible first-line candidate.

All anthracyclines can also produce substantial hair loss which may begin a week after the first injection. The amount of hair actually lost varies from individual to individual and is usually restricted to the scalp, although pubic, armpit and facial hair may also be affected. In almost all cases, the hair grows back completely; regeneration begins 1–2 months after the drug is stopped and the new hair is often curlier and of a lighter shade than the hair that has been lost. Most patients choose to cover their heads with wigs, scarves or hats during the period of hair loss.

L-asparaginase works by depriving cancer cells of an essential food stuff, an amino acid called asparagine. It can produce allergic reactions and, less frequently, inflammation of the liver and pancreas. These allergic reactions are sometimes quite serious and can cause difficulty in breathing, or a puffy face and rashes. Other side-effects include tiredness, loss of appetite, stomach cramps and an increase in the amount of sugar in the blood. The latter effect can simulate diabetes and cause frequent urination and increased thirst. Rarely asparaginase can result in thrombosis by altering the synthesis of many of the proteins involved in the body's coagulation process.

Prednisolone is one of the family of steroids that includes anabolic steroids, which are often used illicitly by some athletes to boost their athletic performance. It is not known exactly how steroids work. Prednisolone is usually given by mouth and can cause stomach problems (particularly superficial ulcers) and high blood pressure due to water retention. In rare cases, steroids can also cause psychiatric difficulties, especially depression and other alterations of mood and thinking. In addition, prednisolone can cause muscle cramps, blurred vision and difficulty in sleeping. In individuals who have diabetes, it raises the levels of sugar in the blood. However, its beneficial action is rapid and it has proven to be of exceptional value in acutely ill patients. It also increases the appetite, which is usually beneficial. The side-effects usually disappear when the drug is discontinued. Recently the Dutch

ALL cooperative group completed a study comparing the efficacy of prednisolone with a related steroid called dexamethasone and concluded that substituting dexamethasone for prednisolone results in a better disease-free survival. This finding requires confirmation by other studies. Dexamethasone also has the advantage of penetrating the central nervous system (CNS) more effectively than prednisolone does.

In a typical treatment plan, vincristine is administered by intravenous (i.v.) injection each week for 5–6 weeks, prednisolone each day for 3–4 weeks, daunorubicin by i.v. injection each day on the first 3 days of the treatment cycle, and L-asparaginase by i.v. or subcutaneous injection each day for 10 days, beginning on day 22 of the treatment cycle.

Most specialists believe that the rate at which leukaemic blast cells are killed in blood and bone marrow is an important prognostic indicator. Remission within 2 weeks of commencing induction therapy predicts a better outcome. As DNA technology is increasingly utilised to monitor progress, it is not unusual to detect disease at the molecular level when conventional remission (clinical and morphological) has been achieved. This is referred to as minimal residual disease. The clinical importance of this, especially in the early stages during induction therapy, is not clear. A few laboratories are now able to (semi) quantify disease at the molecular (subclinical) level. This appears to be useful as an increase in molecular abnormality (usually referred to as increasing transcript numbers) often heralds a clinical and morphological relapse.

Once induction treatment has been completed and normal blood counts are restored, therapy directed at the sanctuary sites (particularly the CNS), and consolidation treatment are begun, usually on an outpatient basis. The former involves administering drugs directly into the cerebrospinal fluid (CSF) that bathes the brain and spinal cord. This is referred to as intrathecal therapy and it is administered by means of a spinal tap. Intrathecal therapy is often combined with radiation therapy to the brain and, usually, to the spinal cord. The drug generally used at this stage is methotrexate, given 6 times at weekly intervals beginning on the first day of brain irradiation. Less often, cytosine arabinoside (Ara-C) is used. It is not clear whether single or multiple agents are preferable, but most specialists use methotrexate alone. When multiple drugs are used, hydrocortisone (a steroid) is added to methotrexate and Ara-C. This combination of intrathecal drugs is often referred to as triple therapy. The main problems that may be encountered with CNS therapy are chemical meningitis, seizures (fits) and, rarely, confusion, all of which are reversible. However, because of recent reports of impaired intelligence in young children treated in such a way, especially when radiotherapy is involved, several centres are exploring alternative treatments, such as giving additional drugs.

Most specialists do not advocate this kind of therapy to the other sanctuary sites such as the testes and ovaries because it may interfere with normal development during puberty. In general, these areas are only treated if they have been shown to be invaded by leukaemic cells.

Radiotherapy, as mentioned above, is another form of intensive treatment occasionally used to kill cancer cells by interfering with their growth. Prior to commencing this treatment, the radiation therapy specialist (radiotherapist) must carry out a number of procedures which will enable him/her to localise the area which needs to be treated. He/she will then formulate the treatment plan after discussions with the technical team, who will advise on selection of the appropriate equipment and calculate the amount of radiation required. It is important to calculate carefully the amount of radiation given because too much is harmful and can even cause cancer (as discussed earlier). Once the treatment plan has been agreed upon, the technique will be tested (simulated) and then several mark(ing)s will be placed on the patient's skin, ensuring that the same areas (volumes) are treated each day. When radiation is used as part of CNS therapy, it is usually necessary to divide the treatment over ten sessions (fractions). The treatment is often aimed at the leukaemic cells in one of the sanctuary sites, the membranous cover surrounding the CNS (meninges). At the usual doses, radiation to the CNS causes few side-effects other than reversible hair loss. However, nausea, skin irritation and drowsiness can occur. Very rarely, radiation may cause cataracts in the lens of the eye.

If radiotherapy is given to other areas, such as the testes and ovaries, the side-effects are quite different. The most serious is damage to the special cells required for reproduction, leading to sterility but not affecting sexual potency. Fortunately, however, the need for this treatment is quite rare.

The next phase of the treatment plan is **consolidation**. Its main objective is to minimize tumour load and its value has been clearly confirmed in children. The benefits in adults are not so clear and are being assessed. A variety of cytotoxic drugs are used, including cyclophosphamide, teniposide (VM-26), Ara-C, daunorubicin, etoposide (VP-16) and prednisolone. Some of these drugs have already been discussed; others will be discussed later.

The last phase of the treatment plan, **maintenance**, usually starts soon after completion of CNS and consolidation therapy, and is continued for 2–3 years on an outpatient basis. The role of maintenance therapy has been fully established in both children and adults with ALL. However, the optimum duration of this treatment depends on the type of induction therapy used, and the question of when maintenance therapy should be discontinued is currently being studied. Most specialists offer this for at least 2 years. The intensity of maintainance therapy should be such that both the bone marrow and the immune system are suppressed to avoid treatment failure.

The drugs most often used for maintenance are 6-mercaptopurine and methotrexate, both of which are usually given by mouth. 6-Mercaptopurine acts by interfering with the synthesis of the building blocks of DNA. It is relatively free of major side-effects; toxicity, when seen, is largely due to the suppression of white blood cell, red blood cell and platelet production. It can also cause abnormal liver function, although this is rare.

Methotrexate, which works by preventing cells from making new DNA by blocking the enzyme dihydrofolate reductase, is absorbed and excreted rapidly by normally functioning kidneys; in patients with impaired kidneys, however, it is very poorly excreted, resulting in higher blood levels of the drug. This may produce serious side-effects ranging from nausea and vomiting to ulceration of the entire gut. For this reason, a specialist will always test a patient's kidney function before prescribing methotrexate. Less often hair loss, skin eruptions, liver damage and even lung damage can occur.

Cyclophosphamide is a very useful drug in the treatment of ALL, AML and a variety of other cancers. It has to be activated by liver enzymes before it can function. It is usually given by i.v. injection but an oral form is also available. Cyclophosphamide is used in very high doses in the preparation of patients for transplantation, which will be discussed later. When used in a conventional dose, it has few side-effects—mainly nausea and vomiting. Rarely it can cause bloody urine (haemorrhagic cystitis). This rare side-effect is dose dependent and the specialist will use an antidote (called mesna) when higher doses of cyclophosphamide are used.

Current treatment programmes result in complete remission in most children with ALL except those in the high risk group. More than 70% of the children in the favourable group are cured. Unfortunately, the results are disappointing in children in the high-risk group (see Table 3.2) and in most adults; less than a third are cured. It is not entirely clear why adults fare so much worse than children, even when their risk status appears to be similar. It is possible that age itself is an important prognostic factor, as in AML, but interestingly, the molecular and biological nature of the ALL in these two populations appears to differ. These differences should be studied further.

The poor results in children in the high risk group and in most adults prompted many specialists to explore the potential of bone marrow transplantation for these patients. The results to date are encouraging. Two new drugs that have been found to be effective are teniposide and etoposide (given i.v. or by mouth). These drugs probably work by interfering with cell synthesis, although their precise mechanism of action is unknown. Both drugs are most effective in ALL, particularly in children. The main side-effects associated with etoposide include gut disturbances, suppression of bone marrow, and hair loss. Although teniposide has fewer side-effects, it can in rare instances result in serious lung toxicity.

Future treatment may also include a variety of drugs referred to as cytokines, for example interferon-alpha and interleukins. These are usually produced by recombinant DNA technology whereby proteins which are identical to those normally found in the human body are synthesised in the laboratory. Clinical studies over the past decade have shown that many of these drugs are useful in the treatment of a variety of cancers. For example, interferon-alpha, which will be discussed in more detail later, has been found to be useful in the treatment of CML; interleukins may have a role in the treatment of kidney (renal) cancer and possibly in the context of blood and bone marrow transplantation.

Recently the haemopoietic growth factors, a family of related drugs, have been synthesised and found to be useful in the treatment of ALL. These drugs, particularly granulocyte-macrophage colony-stimulating factor (GM-CSF) and granulocyte colony-stimulating factor (G-CSF), shorten the time for normal granulocytes to regenerate following chemotherapy. This makes it easier to administer chemotherapeutic drugs in a timely fashion and it reduces the chance of infection by shortening the period of severe neutropenia. Several studies combining such haemopoietic growth factors with chemotherapy have now been completed, particularly in the USA. The outcomes of these studies have been fairly consistent in showing a shorter period of neutropenia, and reduced need for antibiotics and hospital stay, but no beneficial effect on the remission rates or the overall cure rates.

The nausea and vomiting associated with most cytotoxic drugs mentioned above can result in considerable distress and debility. In some instances, the patient may become so distressed as to contemplate stopping any further treatment. Fortunately, progress has been made and new drugs, such as granisetron and ondansetron which have very few side-effects—mainly mild and self-limiting headaches—have proved to be highly effective.

Most patients need to make dietary changes and they will be referred to dietary experts who will help in formulating health-promoting diets. Rarely, some patients may require intravenous feeding, known as total parenteral nutrition (TPN), especially if their nausea and vomiting are severe.

Treatment of AML

Most specialists at present treat patients suffering from AML according to whether the patient is above or below 60 years of age because older patients are less able to withstand the rigours of intensive treatment. There may also be intrinsic biological differences in the leukaemic cells at different ages. It is not unusual for older patients to spend three or four periods in hospital in order to complete treatment within 6 months. The treatment plan usually consists of two phases: initial intensive therapy followed by less intensive treatment. Opinions amongst specialists differ as to the merits of these plans, and some use less intensive regimens over a longer period of time. These issues are currently being addressed in clinical trials. Most intensive treatment plans result in about 80% of patients achieving a complete remission, of which about 35% of patients under the age 60 are cured compared with about 15% of those over the age of 60. Research is underway to determine why the elderly fare comparatively badly.

In the 1950s few patients with AML survived for longer than 3 months, and just 10 years ago only a few patients were expected to live for 5 years. The recent improvement in survival is due to new drugs, improved supportive care and other factors, ranging from better training of specialists to technological advances in the diagnosis and monitoring of the patient's progress.

The most successful induction therapy for younger patients (under 60 years) consists of an anthracycline such as daunorubicin or a related drug such as idarubicin for 2–3 days, in conjunction with Ara-C for 7–10 days. A third drug, usually etoposide, is often added but its merits are not well documented, except in patients with the subtypes M4 and M5. It is possible that by adding a fourth drug, usually 6-thioguanine, the success rate might improve, although this has not been proven. 6-Thioguanine, which is relatively free of side-effects, also works by stopping cells from making DNA (as explained earlier, rapidly multiplying leukaemic cells produce large quantities of DNA).

Ara-C has very few harmful effects and most patients tolerate it very well. At higher doses, which are only occasionally used, it sometimes produces seizures (fits) and tremors, but these are fully reversible. Ara-C acts by preventing cells from making DNA.

Since the fundamental drugs used in the induction phase have remained unchanged for over a decade, it is clear that improved rates of remission must be due to improved supportive care and other factors. More recent experience with idarubicin or mitozantrone instead of daunorubicin show a modest improvement in the remission rates.

In the younger patient, the most important prognostic factors appear to be the karyotype and the ease of achieving remission. Adverse features include a high white blood cell count at diagnosis and an unfavourable karyotype. These prognostic factors remain, regardless of how the relapse is managed.

Adults with AML (unlike those with ALL) rarely harbour in sanctuary sites leukaemic cells that are not killed by induction therapy. Consequently, no prophylaxis (such as CNS therapy) is required. Children more often have leukaemic cells in the CNS so, some specialists prefer to treat the CNS. Because patients with AML subtypes M4 and M5 occasionally develop CNS involvement they require CNS therapy, usually cytotoxic drugs given by the intrathecal route, and radiation therapy.

Recently it has been interesting (and gratifying for researchers!) to witness the entry into clinical trials of novel agents which target specific molecular abnormalities responsible for the leukaemia. Patients with AML subtype M3, who often present with bleeding and thrombosis, are usually placed in studies where they receive high doses of the vitamin A derivative, ATRA (see page 33) prior to conventional induction therapy. Current results reveal that many of these patients achieve remission with ATRA therapy, often without a period of myelosuppression and bone marrow hypoplasia, both of which occur with conventional induction therapy for AML. Most of these ATRA-induced remissions are of a short duration, emphasising the need to treat with conventional induction therapy following ATRA-achieved remission. Conventional therapy should be initiated when patients fail to respond to ATRA.

High dose ATRA works at the level of the mutated gene on chromosome 15 (see Chapter 3). ATRA probably binds to the abnormal protein produced by the mutated gene, altering the function of the protein. When ATRA is used in the high doses which are essential for treating this subtype of AML, a number of unique side-effects are encountered. Most patients experience dry skin and their white blood cell count rises rapidly for a while, occasionally approaching $100 \times 10^9/l$ or more. This, of course, is in contrast to conventional induction therapy in which the counts decrease rapidly and in which bone marrow hypoplasia appears essential for a remission. This unique feature implies that remission has occurred as a consequence of the AML cells becoming differentiated and mature.

About a quarter of all patients who receive ATRA develop the retinoic acid syndrome which consists of fever, low blood pressure, shortness of breath and the development of abnormal lungs (infiltrates). The lining surrounding the heart (the pericardium) can become water-logged (pericardial effusion) in rare instances; this is usually completely reversible.

Following successful induction therapy, all young patients must receive further consolidation therapy. In the past most specialists offered treatment similar to induction therapy but with a modest dose reduction, for example, daunorubicin for 2 days and Ara-C for 5 days.

It is not clear what constitutes ideal consolidation therapy and more and more specialists now offer bone marrow transplantation (BMT) from an HLA identical sibling as consolidation therapy. This and the other forms of BMT, such as autologous BMT, will be discussed in the next chapter. Unlike patients with ALL, those with AML do not appear to benefit from maintenance therapy.

The management of AML in patients who are over 60 remains very difficult and there has been little improvement in outcome with modern treatment. There are many reasons for this. Associated medical conditions are more likely in this age group and many specialists feel that such patients may not withstand the rigours of intensive treatment. Even the relatively fit may not tolerate treatment well. So most specialists do not offer transplantation to patients over 60 years.

There appear to be important biological differences between those under and those over 60 years. Most elderly patients have unfavourable (high risk) type karyotypes and many have a predisposing bone marrow abnormality called myelodysplasia (often termed the myelodysplastic syndrome) which is often characterised by a specific chromosomal abnormality (such as monosomy 7, see Fig. 6.4). Many have a long-standing

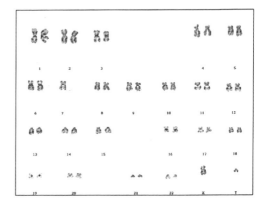

Figure 6.4 A photomicrographic representation of the typical chromosomal abnormality found in patients with a myelodysplastic syndrome, the 7q minus or monosomy 7. (Courtesy of Ms Una Maye, Christie Hospital, Manchester, UK.)

history of anaemias which do not respond to iron or folic acid replacement. It has been established recently that the elderly are also more likely to develop drug resistance as overexpression of the mdr gene is more common in older patients (see page 58 also).

Many studies are exploring the use of haemopoietic growth factors (see page 66) in an attempt to improve supportive care by shortening the period of severe low white blood cell counts. These growth factors also have the potential to enhance chemosensitivity of leukaemic cells by priming them, and they may also decrease drug resistance. Several studies are evaluating this possibility.

It is reasonable to offer conventional therapy to medically fit elderly patients if they are prepared to accept the additional risks and are prepared for a longer hospital stay. On the other hand, there is a good evidence that lower-than-conventional dose therapy, whilst not as effective as conventional dose therapy in producing remissions, may actually offer a similar rate of survival. If a low dose approach is adopted, most specialists will offer oral treatment with drugs like 6-thioguanine, hydroxyurea or etoposide. An oral form of idarubicin has recently entered clinical trials and the initial results appear encouraging, despite fewer complete remissions. Another useful drug which is often employed in this strategy is low-dose Ara-C given subcutaneously.

Treatment of CLL

At present there is no cure for patients who suffer from CLL so most individuals in the early stages of the disease are not treated. If this seems unreasonable, we should remember that more than 2000 years ago, Hippocrates, the great Greek physician, admonished doctors that, above all, they should do no harm to the patient. The remarkable potency of modern drugs makes that advice even more appropriate today. It is therefore not surprising that there are many controversies concerning the treatment of patients with CLL. We and many other specialists feel that it is best to plan treatment in relation to the stage of CLL. This enables one to reach the most rational decision, taking into account the average survival from the time of diagnosis, the likelihood of disease progression, and the likelihood of death from CLL.

Most patients with low-risk CLL (Rai stage 0; see Table 3.4) have an average survival of 10 or more years and most do not die of leukaemia. It would appear best to observe these patients until their disease enters the more aggressive stages when the lymph nodes, liver and spleen are enlarged and when the patient's ability to produce normal numbers of marrow cells—red blood cells, white blood cells and platelets—is impaired. At this stage anaemia, bleeding problems and serious infections may manifest.

The issue of when therapy should be initiated has been explored in a number of well-designed studies which have shown that for patients with low-risk CLL there is no advantage in beginning treatment at the time of diagnosis. When treatment is required, most specialists use chlorambucil which is generally given by mouth and is relatively free of side-effects. Some doctors may add steroids, usually prednisolone. Although this appears to be a useful combination, opinions vary. The main side-effects of chlorambucil are light-headedness and, rarely, rashes.

A promising new drug called fludarabine has been undergoing trials. Improvements in leukaemia treatment are usually made in small steps rather than in giant strides, and each change must be evaluated carefully before it becomes a permanent part of patient care. Trials are usually conducted cooperatively by several centres, often in different countries. Results suggest that fludarabine is a useful drug when the disease is not responding to chlorambucil. Fludarabine is a potent drug with more side-effects than chlorambucil, particularly the severity of bone marrow suppression. It also has a few rare and unique side-effects: it can cause interstitial pneumonia (a diffuse lung infection) and haemolytic anaemia, a condition in which the red cell precursors are destroyed prematurely, resulting in a reduction of the number of circulating red cells. Fludarabine occasionally causes hair loss. Pentostatin (5′-deoxycoformycin), a similar drug, is sometimes used when chlorambucil fails. Another new drug, cladribine, has just entered clinical trials.

Patients with an intermediate-risk CLL (Rai stages I and II; see Table 3.4) have an average survival of about 5 years. The critical issue appears to be the tumour burden. Patients who have few or modest symptoms may not require immediate treatment and a strategy similar to that used for treating low-risk patients can be adopted. This is in contrast to those with moderately severe to severe symptoms and a high tumour burden (large lymph nodes, spleen or liver or very high lymphocyte count) who often require immediate therapy. Most specialists offer chlorambucil first and then, perhaps, fludarabine. The value of combination chemotherapy remains unknown at present as most studies have shown no clear-cut benefit from its use.

Patients with high risk CLL (Rai stages III and IV; see Table 3.4), who have an average survival of 3–4 years, should be offered treatment at the time of diagnosis. These patients have a high probability of developing progressively advancing disease and many will die from the leukaemia. These patients benefit *symptomatically* from chlorambucil. Clinical studies now underway are exploring the advantages of combination chemotherapy and fludarabine over chlorambucil. Interferons, which are discussed on page 74 , have also been assessed but are not particularly useful.

Radiation therapy is occasionally used to relieve symptoms produced by bulky lymph nodes or an enlarged spleen. In the past total-body irradiation was sometimes used but it is now not used because of the resulting bone marrow suppression.

Recently there has been considerable interest in the use of transplants to treat younger patients with high risk CLL. This will be discussed in the next chapter. Combination therapy is often used for treating patients with prolymphocytic leukaemia, usually with cyclophosphamide, adriamycin (similar to daunorubicin), vincristine and prednisolone. Unfortunately, although the initial responses are encouraging, the long-term results are poor.

Most patients with hairy cell leukaemia require treatment. In the past a splenectomy was the initial choice and almost all patients benefited for at least a few months, largely due to fewer infections and lesser blood transfusion requirements. Unfortunately, most develop progressive disease and require other therapies.

Over the past decade several novel approaches have been established as first line therapies for patients with hairy cell leukaemia. Interferons, especially interferon alpha (IFN-α), have resulted in over 90% of all patients showing a substantial benefit. Most patients enjoy long periods of remission, but many relapse when interferon therapy is discontinued. Interferons are a family of protein molecules of biological origin (now synthesised by recombinant DNA technology) with many properties (including antiviral, antiproliferative) which affect the immune system in various ways. They have been available since the 1970s but it was not until the early 1980s that most of their properties became well characterised. They are useful in treating hairy cell leukaemia, and CML (which is discussed in the next section). They may also be useful for treating some types of lymphomas. Interferons are also valuable in managing a number of viral diseases, in particular liver disease caused by the hepatitis B and C viruses.

IFN-α is administered by subcutaneous injection, usually three times a week, but sometimes more often. Early in the treatment nearly all patients experience fevers, muscle aches, joint pains, weakness and lethargy, all of which resemble influenza. These symptoms can be minimized by taking paracetamol or aspirin (or equivalent) 30 min before each injection. Less common side-effects include anorexia, diarrhoea, weight loss and depression. Most patients get used to this drug after 2–3 weeks, and subsequently experience very few side-effects.

Two other very effective drugs in the treatment of hairy cell leukaemia are pentostatin and cladribine, which were mentioned earlier. Current studies suggest that cladribine might be the most effective of the three but formal proof is still awaited.

Patients with ATLL are often treated with combination chemotherapy, similar to that used in treating PLL and related diseases. Nearly all patients respond to this treatment but, unfortunately, most relapse within 6–12 months. A variety of immunological methods of treatment are being assessed, particularly the use of antibodies against specific antigens which are known to play a key role in the development of ATLL.

Treatment of CML

CML has evolved from being incurable to potentially curable by allogeneic haemopoietic stem cell transplantation, but for the present the proportion of patients who do qualify for transplant remains rather small. We will discuss this in the next chapter.

Radiotherapy was the principal palliative treatment for CML until the 1950s when busulphan, a drug which acts by interfering with the ability of the myeloid cells to divide, replaced it. In the early 1980s a related drug, hydroxyurea, became the recommended choice because of its ease of use and lack of potentially serious side-effects. Moreover, clinical studies comparing the use of hydroxyurea to busulphan showed a better survival with hydroxyurea. It is relatively free from side-effects but occasionally nightmares can occur, particularly if the drug is taken at night.

Over the past few years, IFN-α, mentioned in the section on treatment of CLL (page 72), has been found to be the most effective treatment in the early phases of CML, and it appears to offer the possibility of long-term disease control to a small minority of patients. Today IFN-α is the treatment of choice for the initial management of these patients. A number of studies exploring the role of IFN-α in treating patients with CML have now been completed and have confirmed that IFN-α prolongs survival for patients who achieve a major cytogenetic response (a complete or a near complete disappearance of cells bearing the leukaemia-specific Philadelphia chromosome). The results of the UK Medical Research Council study, which was reported in 1995, also showed that a cytogenetic response may not be a prerequisite for benefit from treatment with IFN-α. The optimum dose, duration and route of administration of IFN-α are not obvious but several studies now underway should offer clarification. Specialists are also exploring the possibility of combining IFN-α therapy with other well-established antileukaemic drugs such as Ara-C.

Another approach to treatment involves leucapheresis, the removal of large numbers of white blood cells from a patient's blood by means of a blood cell separator. This allows the specialist to selectively remove selected cellular components of blood, which is useful for treating patients with leukaemias and for collecting particular blood components from healthy blood donors for administration to the patient. Leucapheresis is also useful in managing leukaemia patients when chemotherapy cannot be used with safety, as during pregnancy. It is also useful as an adjunct to chemotherapy in patients whose very high white blood cell counts must be lowered quickly in order to prevent a major catastrophe such as a stroke, which can result from white blood cells blocking major blood vessels of the brain.

In the more aggressive stage of CML, combinations of cytotoxic drugs are usually required, and treatment is similar to that for acute leukaemia. The treatment plan will often depend on whether the leukaemic cells are mainly lymphoid or myeloid. The success rate in treating the aggressive stage of CML, particularly the myeloid forms, is, unfortunately, poor. Some patients with the lymphoid form of disease respond very well for a year or more. The drugs that are most useful include vincristine and prednisolone.

With the elucidation of the molecular abnormalities underlying the pathogenesis of CML, a number of drugs which attempt to inhibit the formation of P210 have been synthesised. One such agent with highly specific activity against BCR-ABL is due to enter clinical trials shortly. Needless to say, novel agents such as this and ATRA, which was discussed earlier, are paving the way for a new era in the treatment of leukaemias. This will be discussed in the final chapter.

7 Blood and bone marrow transplantation

Since the early 1940s, doctors have been interested in replacing diseased bone marrow with healthy marrow, not only because the marrow is a source of cancerous cells (although not the only one) but also because the risk of damage to marrow seriously limits cancer therapy. Many specialists believed that very high doses of chemotherapy drugs would benefit patients with acute leukaemias, but it was impossible to give such doses because of the damage caused to normal bone marrow cells. However, if the patient's marrow, destroyed by high-dose treatment, could be replaced by new marrow, the amount of the drug that could be given would be limited only by its toxicity to other tissues and organs. Extensive experiments in animals showed that this was indeed true. In addition, it was found that is was not necessary to place healthy donor marrow cells directly into a recipient's marrow cavity—these cells could simply be infused into a vein and they would spontaneously find their way to the marrow cavity where they would begin to grow and reproduce. This research paved the way for bone marrow transplantation in man. Donnal Thomas of the Fred Hutchinson Cancer Center, Seattle, USA, was awarded the Nobel Prize in 1990 for his substantial contributions to this research.

In the early 1960s, specialists started to use bone marrow transplantation (BMT) in the treatment of patients with acute leukaemias. However, since the healthy bone marrow came from a person (the host) whose immune and genetic make-up was different from those of the person receiving it (the recipient), serious problems arose from immunological incompatibility. The ideal donor was therefore an identical twin of the recipient because the genes in both twins are identical and therefore no genetic barriers exist. Transplants between identical twins, known as syngeneic transplants, were then and still are (for obvious reasons) rare. However, subsequent

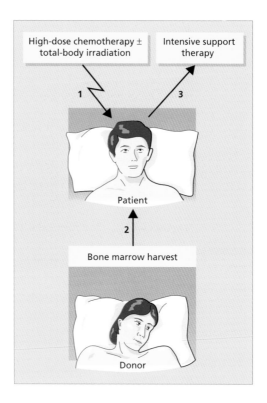

Figure 7.1 Allogeneic BMT schematically represented.

research showed that other family members could also be used as donors, in so-called allogeneic transplants (see Fig. 7.1).

In order to understand how nonidentical family members can be used as donors, it is useful to look at some of the major immunological barriers to BMT. These barriers are determined by a specific set of genes contained in the major histocompatibility complex (MHC) that in turn determines which of the human leucocyte antigens (HLA) a person has. The most important ones are HLA-A, HLA-B, HLA-C, HLA-DR, HLA-DQ and HLA-DP antigens. Without going into detail, there is a 25% chance that any one brother or any sister of a patient will have an HLA make-up identical to the patient and therefore can be a compatible donor. HLA antigens should not be confused with the major blood group antigens (A, B and O), which are very different. Blood group incompatibility is not a major problem in BMT and even if it does occur, it is possible to simply centrifuge (spin down) the collected bone marrow and remove the incompatible red blood cells.

Unfortunately, even when the antigens of the MHC are identical, the acceptance of a bone marrow graft is not guaranteed. The donor's T-lymphocytes can attack the cells of the host because of minor immunological differences between the donor's and the recipient's cells, which are not detected by the tests used at present; these differences can lead to the potentially serious illness of graft-vs-host disease (GVHD). GVHD can produce rashes, severe diarrhoea, liver disturbances, weight loss and, occasionally, serious infections. Graft rejection by the host may also occur if the recipient's lymphocytes destroy the donor's cells.

These perplexing phenomena led to attempts to suppress the recipient's immune system in order to make rejection and other related complications less likely. A variety of approaches were tried and many were indeed found to improve the success rate of the graft substantially. Most treatment regimens now in use involve chemotherapy plus radiotherapy and they are an important part of bone marrow 'conditioning' programmes that provide for the establishment of conditions in which a graft is unlikely to be rejected. A successful conditioning programme should also be able to kill all the leukaemic cells present. Most specialists use high doses of the drug cyclophosphamide followed by high-dose radiotherapy to the whole body (total-body irradiation or TBI), which can be given in a variety of ways.

Whereas measures intended to prevent graft rejection are almost always successful, those designed to overcome GVHD have had limited success until recently. GVHD appears to involve T-lymphocytes of donor origin, and drugs that attack these and other immunologically active cells should reduce the tendency of the graft to reject the host. Two major drugs, cyclosporin A and methotrexate, have been used with variable success. Unfortunately, cyclosporin A can sometimes produce kidney problems which may lead to high blood pressure and water retention and it may also produce hair growth over the entire body (hirsutism); methotrexate is relatively free of toxic effects at the doses used. Other methods which are proving to be successful in eradicating or reducing GVHD are being developed. However, the problem remains of how to attack all leukaemic cells effectively while at the same time coping with GVHD. It is not clear at present why this should be so difficult.

It is important to distinguish between graft rejection and graft failure. The former implies the recognition and subsequent destruction of stem cells by the recipient's T-lymphocytes (and other lymphocytes, such as NK cells) and this can often be overcome by immunosuppression. Graft failure, on the other hand, usually implies that the graft has not 'taken'. This could be due, for example, to an insufficient infusion of stem cells or because the donor's marrow is manipulated (treated) with drugs or antibodies resulting in microenvironment abnormalities. Such difficulties are usually nonimmunological and will not therefore be corrected by increasing immunosuppression. We will discuss these aspects further later in this chapter.

Medical aspects of BMT

Timing

The timing of BMT is extremely important and it depends largely on the nature of the underlying leukaemia. In general, patients with acute leukaemia who are in complete remission, are relatively young (under 50 years of age), have an HLA-identical sibling donor, and who wish to undergo the transplantation procedure are eligible. The transplant is carried out in patients with AML after they have completed consolidation chemotherapy and are in complete remission. At this time, the number of surviving leukaemic cells is likely to be very small. However, for those patients with AML who have 'favourable' risk factors at the time of diagnosis, it is recommended not to perform a transplant but to keep the patient under surveillance after consolidation chemotherapy. Transplantation should be considered after relapse and a second remission. The circumstances in which BMT is most likely to be effective in patients with ALL are still being studied. Current results support the early use of BMT for those patients with ALL who have high risk factors. For all other patients, transplants are reserved for patients who suffer a relapse.

The ideal time for BMT in patients with CML appears to be as soon as the diagnosis has been made while the patient is still in the chronic phase. This can be a problem because most patients feel completely well at this time and many do not want to undergo a potentially fatal treatment. Most patients would prefer to wait until the end of this indolent phase; but, it is clear that the transplant is far less likely to be successful at this stage than in the earlier chronic phase. A reasonable approach is to offer all patients with CML who are under the age of 40 a transplant option as early as possible. For those aged 40–55 years, IFN-α therapy is initiated and if there is no major cytogenetic response after a year or so, a transplant can be contemplated. The autografting option is discussed latter.

Patients with CLL are, in general, not considered for BMT. Less than 5% of patients with CLL are under 50 years of age and it may be useful to consider entering this group into clinical trials exploring the potential of BMT. This appears reasonable in the light of recent preliminary results from a small series of patients with CLL who had a BMT.

Selection of the donor

Standard laboratory tests are carried out to establish the HLA status of a patient's brothers and sisters. If there is still doubt about the identity of HLA genes in the patient and prospective sibling donor, a series of other molecular tests for HLA genes can be undertaken.

As discussed earlier, the chance of any one sibling being an identical match at the HLA-A, B, and DR levels is 25%. It is most unlikely that either of the parents will be a complete match since each person inherits one of two possible paternal and one of two possible maternal chromosome sets to make up its HLA type. In general, if the average number of siblings in a family is just over two, the probability of identifying a potential donor is actually about 30%. These constraints obviously limit the number of potential donors considerably. The lack of an HLA identical sibling donor for a patient whose only chance of survival is to have BMT has inspired specialists to try to find acceptable family member donors who are not genetically HLA identical. Recently, we and others have also been using HLA-matched unrelated donors, and the early results are encouraging. Current data suggest a 50% probability of finding a matched unrelated donor. This and the (modest) success achieved by others performing BMTs using matched unrelated donors has led to several international computerised registries for storing HLA-typing data. For example, in the UK the Anthony Nolan Bone Marrow Trust, a registry with data on nearly 300 000 potential marrow donors, has been in operation since the 1970s. As the number of available marrow donors increases, we can anticipate a higher chance of finding a suitable donor.

What happens to the donor?

The donor is usually admitted to the hospital on the day before the marrow is to be harvested (collected). At this time, he or she will be examined thoroughly and an anaesthetist will make sure there are no problems in giving the patient a general anaesthetic. Bone marrow is collected from the hip and sometimes also the breast bone while the donor is anaesthetised, as described on page 47 (Fig. 4.6). For a successful graft, about 1 litre of normal healthy marrow is needed, which usually takes about 60–90 min to collect. Figure 7.2 shows bone marrow being harvested.

In order to prevent the donor from becoming anaemic, a blood transfusion is normally given during the procedure. Usually, the blood transfused is the donor's own blood which was taken about 2 weeks earlier. This is termed an *autologous* transfusion; it not only avoids unnecessary demands on the blood bank but also, and more importantly, avoids the risks, minimal though they are, associated with transfusions from other people, such as hepatitis or HIV infection. The only real risks to the donor are those associated with having a general anaesthetic. Pain at the harvest site is unusual. It is important to emphasise that there is no permanent loss of marrow function for the donor, since the bone marrow regenerates fully in a few weeks.

However, psychological effects pertaining to marrow donation are not uncommon. Some donors may feel guilty if the recipient does not do well following BMT; others may feel rejected if initial tests suggest that they may be potential donors but the subsequent tests identify a more suitable donor

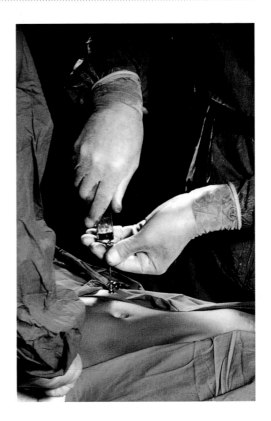

Figure 7.2 Bone marrow being harvested (collected). (Courtesy of Dr. Godfrey Morgenstern, Christie Hospital, Manchester, UK.)

within the family. It is important for all donors to realise that the success or failure of BMT is totally unrelated to recognisable characteristics of the donor.

Once the marrow has been harvested, it is stored in plastic bags with anticoagulant to prevent clotting. The marrow will contain tiny chips of bone, and some clumps of cells; these will be filtered out using a series of fine meshes. The marrow is then placed in a plastic pack and is ready to be given to the recipient. Before the transplant, the marrow may be treated with a variety of agents, such as monoclonal antibodies, designed to remove the T-lymphocytes. It is important to emphasise again that there is no permanent loss to the donor.

What happens to the recipient?

In most BMT centres, the recipient is admitted about 2 weeks before the transplant is due. Patients are admitted to single isolation rooms which are specially designed to provide an environment that is as free as possible of germs to reduce the risk of airborne infections, which can be dangerous in the first few weeks after BMT. After a thorough physical examination, a catheter (usually a Hickman catheter; see page 56 and Fig. 6.1) is inserted into one of the patient's veins to provide easy access to the circulation. As discussed earlier, many specialists also use these catheters during the initial treatment of patients with acute leukaemia.

The patient is then started on a conditioning regimen involving high-dose chemotherapy and radiation therapy as outlined earlier. This is designed to eradicate the leukaemic cells and to cause immunosuppression in order to minimize the chances of the bone marrow graft being rejected. The precise details of the drug and radiation programmes used vary from centre to centre and also with the type of leukaemia being treated. Conditioning is followed by the infusion of the donor marrow, after which technical aspects of the BMT procedure are complete and the supportive phase begins.

The period of BMT

Following the transplant, all patients stay in isolation rooms for about 4 weeks and most need intensive nursing care for the first 15 days. As a direct result of the conditioning procedure, patients develop a marked reduction in all of their blood cells (pancytopenia) which lasts for about 2 weeks, until the donor marrow cells have grown (engrafted) and begun to produce blood cells. During the pancytopenic period, the patient is at a very high risk of infection and will also have profound anaemia and thrombocytopenia which will necessitate blood and platelet transfusions. All blood products transfused after the transplant are irradiated in order to destroy the T-lymphocytes they contain and thus prevent some of these cells from attacking the cells of the patient. The remaining blood cells are not destroyed by this irradiation.

To safeguard against infections, all patients receive intravenous antibiotics which are effective against a wide range of organisms, as well as antiviral and antifungal agents given by mouth. The antibiotics are stopped when the patient's new marrow has generated at least 500 granulocytes per microlitre, provided there is no evidence of an infection. Occasionally, intravenous antifungal drugs such as amphotericin B will also be required to prevent serious fungal infection. The severe immune deficiency which may persist for long periods (up to 2 years), predisposes the patient to viral infection, a serious problem despite the increasing use in most BMT centres of protective oral antiviral agents.

Many BMT centres are exploring the use of haemopoietic growth factors (see page 66). These are used to hasten the production of blood cells during the period after BMT. By shortening the time for the recovery of granulocyte formation the risks of infection are reduced.

During the first 10 days following transplant, most patients will develop mouth ulcers which make eating difficult, and they will therefore need special nutritional care. Furthermore, patients use up their own body protein (principally from muscle) during this period because the conditioning regimen causes the tissues to use enormous quantities of energy. Most centres provide diets of 2000–3000 calories a day, consisting of freshly cooked foods containing few bacteria. In addition, the majority of patients need intravenous feeding (TPN). Good nutrition is important because malnutrition is itself immunosuppressive.

It is not uncommon at this stage to encounter psychological problems ranging from anxiety related to the transplant procedure and lack of social contact while in isolation, to severe claustrophobia and dependency. To minimize these effects, social contact is allowed during the isolation period as long as it complies with the rules of reverse barrier nursing. This requires the visitors (as well as the medical staff) to be 'isolated' from the patient by wearing a gown, gloves, face mask and often a hat. This is done in order to reduce the chances of the patient acquiring an infection. Most partners and parents want, and are given, unlimited access to a patient's room.

The post-transplant period involves considerable disruption and often requires the entire family to change its life style. However, the difficulties are acceptable when the outcome is successful. Most families must plan for at least one member to arrange to stay near the patient for at least 3 months. Transplant teams usually include social workers, clinical psychologists and psychiatrists who can be very helpful in supporting the family.

Towards the end of the first month after transplant, most patients are in good condition, with blood counts approaching normal, and they are allowed to leave the hospital. However, their immune system remains defective and will not return to normal for up to 2 years. It is therefore important for the continued success of the transplant to maintain very close medical follow-up of all patients, usually with weekly or fortnightly outpatient visits for the first 6 months.

The most serious complications which may arise during the 6 months after the transplant are lung inflammation (interstitial pneumonia) and GVHD. The lung condition is a result of the combined effects of GVHD, previous chemotherapy, radiation therapy given as part of the conditioning regimen, and viral infections. One particular viral infection, due to cytomegalovirus (CMV), is especially important. Currently, there is no totally reliable treatment of CMV infection but ganciclovir is usually effective in suppressing or eradicating CMV infection. They unquestionably decrease the incidence of other viral infections such as those due to *Herpes simplex* (cold sores) and *Herpes zoster* (chickenpox-related) infections.

Nevertheless, the overall incidence of lung inflammation is 10–20% and, sadly, most of the patients who acquire it will die. Lack of specific treatment for this grave complication means that we are restricted to supportive care only, in an attempt to buy time to enable the patient's immune system to recover enough to be able to guard against infection.

GVHD has been less of a problem since it became possible to remove T-lymphocytes from donor marrow. The most common effects are on the skin and lining of the gut, but the liver is also occasionally affected. When GVHD appears within a hundred days of transplantation, it is termed acute, while GVHD that comes on more than 100 days after the transplantation procedure is known as chronic. It has, however, been observed that when T-lymphocytes are removed from donor marrow, the rate of relapse increases although the risk of GVHD is diminished. It has now been established that this increase in the relapse rate is due to the loss of the so-called 'Graft Versus Leukaemia' (GVL) effect. Specialists are currently exploring the extent(s) to which the donor allograft should be depleted of the T-lymphocytes in an attempt to optimise a balance in which the risk of GVHD is lowered without compromising the GVL effect; they are also studying the potential role of cytokines such as interleukin-2. Interestingly the importance of the GVL reaction appears to be particularly instrumental in the outcome of BMT in patients with CML.

Acute GVHD occurs in about 25% of cases and is a serious complication, which can be fatal. Current treatment, usually with high-dose steroids and cyclosporin A, is rather unsatisfactory. Chronic GVHD also occurs in about 25% of transplant patients, and generally affects the skin and the lining of the mouth; on rare occasions the intestine and the lung are involved. Treatment is a little more successful than for the acute form and consists of low-dose steroids and immunosuppressive agents such as azathioprine. Because these drugs predispose to infection, broad-spectrum antibiotics are also given.

By the end of the 6 month period following BMT, most successfully transplanted patients are able to go back to work. They are usually seen about once a month at their local hospital and about four times a year at their transplant centre. After about 2 years, when the immune system is expected to have recovered, a programme of re-immunisation with inert or killed vaccines (live vaccines must *never* be given to a BMT patient) can be started. This is because all previously acquired immunity will have been destroyed by the transplant procedure.

Unfortunately, relapse is a serious problem in all types of leukaemia, most often within the first 2 years after the transplant. However, after this, the risk gradually decreases to become minimal after about 5 years, with the major exception of patients with CML who may relapse after years of leukaemia-free survival. This is in keeping with the natural history of CML and its slow evolution (see pages 74–75). Patients with acute leukaemia can be confidently assumed to be cured after 8 years. The risk of leukaemic relapse following transplantation for AML seems to be higher in people older than 40 years and in those with poor prognostic features such as a high white blood cell count at the time of diagnosis.

Most patients who survive for 5 years or more following a BMT enjoy excellent health and most are able to pursue a lifestyle which they had enjoyed prior to having been diagnosed. The European Group for Blood and Marrow Transplantation (EBMT) recently published their findings of nearly 800 patients who had been transplanted prior to 1985 and had survived at least 5 years. The group observed that whilst over 90% of all patients had a productive and good quality life, some still faced the prospects of illness and even death. The chief causes of death were the relapse of their leukaemia, development of a second cancer (causally related to the treatment received) and chronic GVHD. Most second cancers seem to affect the skin and are usually easily cured by surgery. Rarely, cancers of the airways and oesophagus (gut) develop, resulting in death.

Specialists have also reported an increased risk of lymphomas, usually within 2–3 years of the transplant. Many of these lymphomas appear to be causally associated with EBV infection in donor cells (see Chapter 2). Some of these lymphomas also appear to be associated with the immunosuppressive treatment and they often regress when this treatment is discontinued.

The results of bone marrow transplantation in leukaemia

AML

Up until early 1970, BMT was used in AML only after the failure of all other treatments. Then, between 1970 and 1975, American specialists were able to show that a small proportion of patients with advanced AML, which was resistant to all conventional treatments, became long-term survivors when treated with BMT from HLA-identical sibling donors. This led many experts to speculate that better results might be achieved if BMT were carried out while the patient was in first complete remission, and therefore most leukaemia centres throughout the world now offer BMT to patients who are in first remission. Current analysis of the results of this form of treatment suggest that the cure rate is nearly 50%. The chances of a cure in the second remission have appeared to be less good, although a recent study indicates that they might be comparable.

With chemotherapy alone, 80% of patients achieve complete remission, but only 35% of those under the age of 60 achieve a cure; in children under 15 years of age, almost 60% remain in complete remission after 3 years, but it is not yet known how many of these will relapse subsequently. This is why BMT has become routine in many centres provided that the patient is relatively young (most centres have an upper age limit of 50 years), has an HLA-identical sibling donor, and wants the transplant. It should, however, be noted that further progress is being made with a variety of chemotherapeutic drugs and it is likely that the results with chemotherapy alone will improve further; this will make it difficult to choose between further chemotherapy and BMT once complete remission is achieved. However, despite the risks, at present BMT offers the best chance of cure in AML. The question of when to transplant a patient with AML has not yet been convincingly answered and is being addressed in several current studies.

ALL

Chemotherapy has been highly successful in the treatment of childhood ALL and cure rates of 60–80% are being obtained in the most favourable groups of patients. About 35% of adults who have a good prognosis, i.e. those who are between 15 and 20 years old, with a low white blood cell count, minor degrees of organ enlargement, and no evidence of CNS involvement, are cured. As a result, the role of BMT for such patients has not been looked at very carefully.

For the considerable number of adult patients with ALL who have a poor prognosis, the probability of a cure with chemotherapy alone is relatively small. These patients, and others who relapse after primary treatment, should probably receive BMT if a suitable donor is available. Current results show that about 30% of patients with ALL transplanted in the second or later remission are cured.

CML

It has become clear, especially over the last 5 years, that BMT offers the best chance of curing CML in the chronic phase of the disease, when the cure rate approaches 60–70%. The cure rate of those patients who are transplanted in the later stages falls to 20%, and the chance of relapse is 50% compared with less than 10% for those transplanted in the chronic phase. Patients with CML who have a compatible donor should either be transplanted in the chronic phase or not at all.

There are still a number of important questions that remain unresolved in relation to BMT for CML. For example, it is still uncertain whether or not the spleen should be removed at the time of the transplant; the best time for BMT during the chronic phase is still uncertain. These and other problems are being carefully studied.

Autologous BMT

Although allogeneic BMT is most promising for the treatment of certain subtypes of acute leukaemia and CML, unfortunately it is not available to most patients because of a lack of suitable donors. This has led to attempts to use the patient's own bone marrow cells. This technique is called autografting and the idea behind it is fairly simple (Fig. 7.3). Bone marrow cells are harvested under general anaesthesia from the hip bone of the patient. Usually approximately 1 litre of marrow is aspirated, a loss which does not harm the patient, as the marrow cells usually regenerate quickly. The harvested marrow cells can be stored for up to 54 h at 4°C or they can be frozen in liquid nitrogen to be used up to 6 years later.

In acute leukaemias, the marrow cells are harvested during the period of rapid recovery following a course of intensive chemotherapy. During this period, the residual leukaemic cell population will have been reduced as near to zero as possible and after further intensive treatment the marrow cells are infused into a vein. Some specialists perform this procedure twice, the marrow cells being harvested for the second time in the recovery phase after the first autograft. This procedure is called a 'double autograft' and may yield slightly better results than a 'single autograft'.

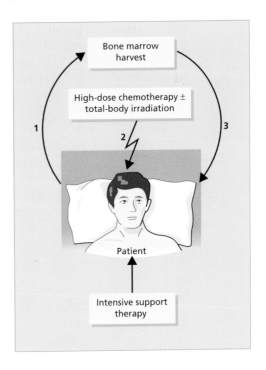

Figure 7.3 Autologous BMT schematically represented.

Although this technique is not difficult to perform, the marrow that is removed may contain leukaemic cells which escaped destruction by the chemotherapy. A possible solution is to treat the collected marrow cells in such a way that only the leukaemic cells are destroyed and then return the normal marrow to the patient. Several methods have been used to remove leukaemic cells selectively from marrow. These so-called 'purging' techniques are still being evaluated but the most successful methods so far are physical (exploiting the physical differences between the leukaemic and normal marrow cells), immunological (using antibodies to seek out and destroy leukaemic cells), and pharmacological (using drugs which selectively destroy leukaemic cells).

Autologous BMT is not complicated by the problems associated with acute GVHD, and lung inflammation occurs less frequently. Infections are also easier to manage since the immunosuppression is less profound and less prolonged than that which occurs with allogeneic BMT. Recent results have shown a leukaemic free survival at 3 years of up to 50% after autologous BMT of patients with AML in their first complete remission. The 3-year leukaemia free survival for patients with ALL who are transplanted in first complete remission is around 30%. These results are comparable to those obtained with allogeneic BMT, despite the lack of a GVL effect in autologous BMT. It is speculated that as novel approaches to induce GVL effects in autologous transplants are improved, the results should improve further.

Autografting of patients with CML has produced some interesting results. In the 1970s autologous stem cells were collected from the blood or marrow of untreated patients and used a number of years later after intensive treatment of these patients. Some patients recovered normal haemopoiesis for variable periods. We and others have observed that patients with CML who were autografted have prolonged survivals, though the probability of cure is extremely small. With the availability of novel agents with high specificity against BCR-ABL (see page 40), the pretreatment of the autografts with this agent before it is infused into the patient has sound conceptual appeal and is currently being studied. At present, however, treatment of patients with CML with autologous BMT remains under investigation, and research over the next few years will determine its eventual role.

Peripheral blood stem cell transplants

It has been found recently that if marrow cells are made to enter the blood and are then collected and used as an autograft, they are capable of inducing haemopoiesis as efficiently as bone marrow cells harvested from the bone marrow. This procedure, which is called 'peripheral blood stem cell (PBSC) transplant', seems to have two distinct advantages over autologous BMT. First, the recovery (engraftment) appears to be faster; second, it is believed that PBSC may be less contaminated by residual leukaemic cells than bone marrow cells and there may therefore be a greater potential for success. This has not yet been proved. It has been shown that if patients are pretreated with haemopoietic growth factors, the yield of PBSC is substantially increased. Blood cell separa-

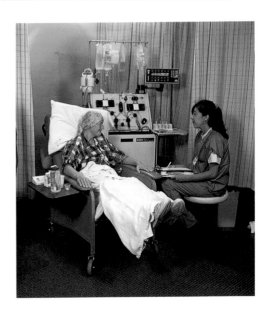

Figure 7.4 A blood cell separator. (Courtesy of Mr Edward Wood, Cobe Laboratories, Lakewood, Colorado, USA.)

tors, such as the Cobe Spectra (Fig. 7.4), are furnished with automated programmes, which facilitate the efficient collection of PBSC.

Over the past few years the transplantation of allogeneic PBSC (now more commonly referred to as peripheral blood progenitor cells (PBPC)) instead of bone marrow cells has become increasingly popular, and a number of studies are comparing these two sources of the transplant (blood vs marrow). Allogeneic PBPC transplantation from HLA-matched donors results in faster engraftment and the need for fewer blood transfusions without a greater incidence of acute or chronic GVHD. Haemopoietic growth factors can safely be given to healthy donors in order to mobilise their stem cells from the marrow to the blood. This technology has already seen a widespread use of autologous PBPC, particularly in patients with lymphomas and breast cancers. Breast cancer is in fact today the most frequent indication for such a transplant in the USA.

An interesting alternative source of allogeneic haematopoietic stem cells is the use of cells collected from the umbilical cord of neonates. The first successful transplantation using cord blood cells was carried out by Elaine Gluckman and her colleagues in Paris, in 1988. Since then, over 300 such transplants using cord blood stem cells have been carried out and cord blood from unrelated donors has been studied recently. There are two important features which make cord blood (especially from unrelated donors) particularly attractive as a source of stem cells for transplantation in patients who lack an HLA-identical donor. First, the immaturity of the haematopoietic stem cells in cord blood may allow engraftment with fewer cells than are required with blood and marrow sources. Secondly, the risk of both acute and chronic GVHD appears less, possibly because of the relative immaturity of cord blood T-lymphocytes. This may permit a greater degree of flexibility than do blood or marrow with regards to HLA differences between the donor and recipient.

8 Future prospects

There is no doubt that enormous advances in our understanding of human cancers have been made in the past decade, and in many ways the study of leukaemia illustrates this trend. Fortunately, this better understanding of cancer has led to an improvement in the treatment of many patients with leukaemia. This is exemplified by the way in which new agents have been developed to target specific molecular abnormalities responsible for the leukaemia. ATRA, a vitamin A derivative, is increasingly being used. ATRA targets the molecular abnormality involving the retinoic acid receptor in acute promyelocytic leukaemia (AML subtype M3). Molecular therapy targeting key enzymes, such as tyrosine kinase, is now entering clinical trials. For example, use of an agent with specific activity against the BCR-ABL tyrosine kinase in chronic myeloid leukaemic has begun. We are undoubtedly now in the era of molecular medicine and can confidently anticipate further novel approaches to targeting various molecular abnormalities.

Our understanding of the bone marrow microenvironment is increasing and it is possible that the future will bring new techniques such as the use of antibodies specifically directed against the products of the abnormal genes to destroy or inactivate leukaemic cells.

Genetic engineering, which allows researchers to pluck genes from chromosomes, has facilitated gene therapy and allowed us to replace defective or missing genes or to add helpful genes. Bone marrow is an ideal candidate for gene therapy as it can be manipulated easily *ex vivo* (outside of the body) and then returned to the recipient. The selection of the haematopoietic stem cells (also known as CD34 positive cells) provides one with a method of isolating the potential targets of gene therapy, the progenitors and stem cells. Gene therapy has proven successful in treating children with severe combined immune deficiency (SCID) in which a key enzyme is missing due to the lack of the pertinent gene. The missing gene can be replaced. As the various technical hurdles are cleared and we unravel the genetic basis of leukaemia further, gene therapy may find an important place.

We have had reasonable success in treating patients with low-risk ALL, particularly children, in whom a cure rate of around 70% can now be anticipated. More recently, a similar order of success has also been achieved by allogeneic BMT in treating patients with CML. Nevertheless, therapy in patients with AML and high-risk ALL, remains difficult and a cure rate of only about 25% is possible at present.

Overall, the treatment of acute leukaemias is difficult to administer and is fairly toxic to the patient, but this should improve as drugs which are safer and more effective in killing leukaemic cells but less likely to damage normal cells are developed. Supportive care is also improving and this will help us deal with some treatment-related complications more promptly and efficiently.

BMT, both allogeneic and autologous, has become fairly well established in the treatment of acute and chronic leukaemias, although it is still surrounded by several controversies. In particular, there is ongoing debate about the best time to perform transplantation. This is particularly difficult when transplanting patients with CML and, perhaps, ALL. The recommendation for BMT in a patient suffering from acute leukaemia depends on several factors, including careful assessment of both the prognosis and the available chemotherapeutic options. Furthermore, family support is crucial to the success of both chemotherapy and BMT.

We have witnessed an enormous increase in the use of peripheral blood stem cell transplants (particularly autologous transplants) and it is very likely that this will be the preferred transplant option when an autologous transplant is indicated. Extensive studies are also exploring the merits of allogeneic PBPC. We are seeking novel ways to increase the availability of BMT by increasing the sources of stem cells, particularly by increasing the pool of matched unrelated donors and, more recently, umbilical cord blood.

For the moment, we can say that the increasing worldwide interest in biology and medicine and the enormous activity occurring in the field of molecular biology make it probable that many forms of blood cancer which are now lethal will be prevented or cured within the next two or three decades.

Glossary

Acute A disease described as acute is of short duration or rapid onset. The term does not imply severity.

Acute lymphoblastic leukaemia (ALL) The most dramatic form of acute leukaemia, which most commonly affects children.

Acute myeloid leukaemia (AML) The most common form of acute leukaemia in adults.

AIDS A life threatening disease caused by HIV-1 and characterised by the breakdown of the body's immune system.

ALL See Acute lymphoblastic leukaemia.

Allogeneic transplant A transplant between individuals other than identical twins.

AML See Acute myeloid leukaemia.

Amphotericin A powerful anti-fungal drug sometimes administered when a patient is immunosuppressed.

Anorexia Loss of appetite for food.

Antibody A protein molecule secreted by B-lymphocytes in response to an antigen.

Antigen A substance that is recognized by the body as foreign.

Apoptosis The body's ability to self-destruct (cell suicide).

Ara-C See Cytosine arabinoside.

Asparaginase An anti-cancer drug given as part of the initial treatment of ALL.

ATL Adult T-cell leukaemia/lymphoma, a disease associated with HTLV-I infection.

ATRA All-trans-retinoic acid, a vitamin A derivative useful in the treatment of acute promyelocytic leukaemia.

Autografting The technique by which a patient's own blood or bone marrow is harvested and later returned; the stem cells are referred to as 'autologous'.

Autologous BMT See Autografting.

Azathioprine An immunosuppressive agent used to treat GVHD.

B-lymphocytes Lymphocytes originating in the bone marrow.

Biological response modifiers Newer anti-cancer drugs, such as interferon, produced by recombinant DNA technology.

Blast cell Primitive blood cells appearing in large numbers in leukaemic bone marrow.

Blast crisis The transition of CML from a chronic to a very aggressive phase.

BMT Bone marrow transplantation.

Burkitt's lymphoma A particular type of cancer; in Africa it is associated with the Epstein–Barr virus.

Busulphan An anti-cancer drug used in the early stage of CML.

Cell cytoplasm The contents of a cell, other than its nucleus.

Cell membrane The outer 'skin' of a cell.

Cell nucleus The central organ of a cell that contains the information it needs to reproduce.

Chemotherapeutic agent A drug used to treat a sickness; most commonly used to refer to an anti-cancer drug.

Chlorambucil A cytotoxic drug often used to treat CLL.

Chromosome 'Strings' of DNA in the nuclei of cells consisting of genes.

Chronic lymphocytic leukaemia The most common type of leukaemia overall, mainly affecting older people.

Chronic myeloid leukaemia Leukaemia characterised by an initial insidious or chronic phase usually followed by an abrupt transition to an aggressive form.

Cladribine A new drug effective for the treatment of hairy cell leukaemia.

CLL See Chronic lymphocytic leukaemia.

CML See Chronic myeloid leukaemia.

CMV See Cytomegalovirus.

Combination chemotherapy Chemotherapy involving more than one drug.

Combined modality treatment Cancer treatment involving drugs and radiation therapy.

Consolidation therapy The second phase of treatment of ALL, given when remission is achieved.

Cord blood transplants Use of haematopoietic stem cells from an umbilical cord for transplantation.

Cyclophosphamide A cytotoxic drug.

Cyclosporin A An immunosuppressive drug sometimes used to treat GVHD.

Cytokines Molecules that the body produces in response to viral and bacterial infection. These molecules assist in the orderly operation of the body's defence responses and include such proteins as interferons and interleukins.

Cytomegalovirus A herpes group virus that is particularly dangerous after BMT.

Cytosine arabinoside A drug sometimes given as part of induction therapy in AML.

Cytotect A drug used to treat CMV.

Cytotoxic Cell-killing drug, usually applied to drugs that kill cells capable of undergoing division.

Daunorubicin An antibiotic given in the initial stages of treatment of ALL and AML.

Deoxyribonucleic acid The genetic material present in every cell.

DNA See Deoxyribonucleic acid.

EBV See Epstein–Barr virus.

Epirubicin A drug similar to daunorubicin but with fewer adverse effects.

Epstein–Barr virus A virus implicated in the development of Burkitt's lymphoma.

Erythrocytes The (red) blood cells which are responsible for carrying oxygen and carbon dioxide to and from the lungs.

Etoposide A cytotoxic drug sometimes given to high-risk ALL patients and to patients with AML.

Fludarabine A promising new drug which is effective in advanced CLL.

G-CSF See Granulocyte colony-stimulating factor.

Ganciclovir An anti-viral drug used to treat CMV infections.

Gene The basic unit of inheritance.

Genetic engineering The technology which allows researchers to pluck genes from the chromosomes, or to insert genes.

Gene therapy The replacement of defective or missing genes or the addition of useful genes by means of genetic engineering.

GM-CSF See Granulocyte-macrophage colony-stimulating factor.

Graft-versus-host disease An adverse reaction to a bone marrow graft as a consequence of the recipient T-lymphocytes recognising the donor T-lymphocytes.

Graft-versus-leukaemia A beneficial reaction between donor T-lymphocytes and recipient's leukaemic cells.

Granisetron A drug that prevents or reduces nausea and vomiting.

Granulocyte A type of leucocyte that ingests and destroys foreign bodies.

Granulocyte colony-stimulating factor A haemopoietic growth factor that has been found useful in the treatment of ALL.

Granulocyte-macrophage colony-stimulating factor A haemopoietic growth factor that has been found useful in the treatment of ALL.

Haemopoiesis (also Haematopoiesis) The process of blood cell development and differentiation.

Haemopoietic growth factors A family of biological agents which have been found to be useful in the treatment of ALL.

HLA See Human leucocyte antigens.

HTLV See Human T-cell lymphotropic virus.

Human leucocyte antigens (HLA) The major factors determining compatibility between bone marrow donors and recipients.

Human T-cell lymphotropic virus A virus implicated in certain kinds of leukaemia.

Hydroxyurea A cytotoxic drug used to treat CML.

Idarubicin A drug similar to daunorubicin, but with fewer adverse side-effects.

Immune deficiency Inadequacy in the body's natural protective mechanisms.

Immunosuppression The process of 'damping down' a patient's immune system to prevent graft rejection.

Immunotherapy Treatment to stimulate or restore the ability of the immune system.

Induction therapy Initial therapy designed to eliminate all evidence of leukaemia.

Interferon A family of biological agents which appears to be effective against some forms of leukaemia.

Interleukin A cytokine which has been found to be useful in kidney (renal) cancer. It is possible that it may also have a role in blood and bone marrow transplantation.

Leucapheresis The selective removal of large numbers of white blood cells from a patient's blood by means of a blood cell separator.

Leucocytes The (white) blood cells responsible for combating infection and destroying alien material.

Leukaemia Blood cancer; literally 'white blood'.

Lymphocytes Types of leucocytes that may secrete substances to destroy invading organisms.

Maintenance phase The phase of leukaemia treatment that takes place when most of the leukaemic cells have been killed; better described as continuation treatment.

Major histocompatibility complex The specific set of genes that determine an individual's HLA status.

6-Mercaptopurine A drug used in ALL maintenance chemotherapy.

Metastasis The passage of malignant cells around the body from their site of origin to establish new cancers elsewhere.

Methotrexate An anti-cancer drug usually given in the later stages of treatment for ALL.

MHC See Major histocompatibility complex.

Mitozantrone A cytotoxic drug like daunorubicin but with fewer adverse side-effects.

Mixed lymphocyte reactivity A test carried out to select a potential bone marrow donor from a group of compatible relatives.

MLR See Mixed lymphocyte reactivity.

Monocyte A type of leucocyte.

Oncogene Activated form of a proto-oncogene that is directly involved in causing malignant growth.

Ondansetron A drug that prevents or reduces nausea and vomiting.

Pancytopenia A reduction in all the cellular elements (red blood cells, white blood cells, platelets) of the blood to below normal levels.

PBPC Peripheral blood progenitor cells—also known as CD34 positive stem cells—which are most important for blood and marrow transplants.

Pentostatin A useful drug for treating CLL and PLL.

Philadelphia chromosome An abnormal chromosome in the leukaemic cells of most patients with CML.

PLL Prolymphocytic leukaemia; a variety of CLL.

Plasma The fluid part of the blood in which the blood cells float.

Platelet See Thrombocyte.

Prednisolone Steroid drug used as part of combination chemotherapy.

Primary tumour The mass of cells (a tumour) which is at the original site of a cancer.

Prophylaxis Preventive treatment.

Proto-oncogene Genes which have the ability to lead to a disturbed growth pattern which can in turn lead to a malignant growth. They are made up of sequences of DNA which are susceptible to mutation.

Purging techniques Methods of selectively removing leukaemic cells from bone marrow.

Radiation therapy The use of radiation (high energy X-rays) to kill cancer cells.

Red blood cells See Erythrocytes.

Relapse Recurrence of a disease following remission.

Remission The temporary disappearance of the signs and symptoms of a disease.

Retrovirus A virus which may be involved in causing some types of cancer.

Reverse barrier nursing Nursing techniques designed to protect a patient from infection.

Ribonucleic acid A messenger substance which carries genetic information within a cell.

RNA See Ribonucleic acid.

Sanctuary sites Areas of the body which are difficult for anti-leukaemic drugs to reach.

Secondary tumour A tumour which develops as a result of metastasis somewhere other than at the original site of cancer.

Spinal fluid The fluid surrounding the brain and spinal cord.

Spinal tap The technique by which spinal fluid can be sampled or drugs are added (to the spinal fluid).

Stem cell Early cells from which all other blood cells develop.

Supportive therapy Treatment to counter the adverse effects of anti-cancer therapy and to otherwise support the patient.

Syngeneic transplant Transplant between identical twins.

T-lymphocyte A type of lymphocyte processed in the thymus gland.

Telomerase An enzyme which is involved in the body's control system that tells cells to stop dividing after a certain time. If this control is suppressed, cells multiply out of control and cancer may arise.

Teniposide A new, experimental anti-cancer drug.

6-Thioguanine A drug sometimes used as part of induction therapy in AML.

Thrombocyte A blood cell responsible for blood clotting; also called platelet.

Tissue-typing The process of finding a suitable (bone marrow) donor for a particular recipient.

Total parenteral nutrition Nutrition given intravenously because a patient cannot feed normally.

TPN See Total parenteral nutrition.

Tumour Literally a swelling, but commonly used to mean a mass of cancer cells.

Vincristine A potent cytotoxic drug given in the early stages of treatment for ALL.

White blood cells See Leucocytes.

Appendices

1 Useful contacts for further help and information

UK

BACUP, 3 Bath Place, London EC2 3JR
  Tel: 0800 181199, 0171 613212
Cancerlink, 17, Britannia House, London WC1X 9JN
  Tel: 0171 8332451
Cancer Relief Macmillan Fund, 15–19 Britten Street, London
  SW3 3TZ
  Tel: 0171 3517811
The Leukaemia Care Society, 14 Kingfisher Court, Exeter EX4 8JN
  Tel: 01392 464848
The Malcolm Sargent Cancer Fund for Children, 14 Abingdon
  Road, London W8 6AF
  Tel: 0171 9374548
Marie Curie Cancer Care, 28 Belgrave Square, London SW1X 8QG
  Tel: 0171 2353325
Leukaemia Research Fund, 43 Great Ormond Street, London
  WC1N 3JJ
  Tel: 0171 4050101

USA

Leukemia Society of America, 600 Third Avenue, New York,
  NY10016
  Tel: 1-800-955-4LSA, 212 5738484
American Cancer Society
  Tel: 1-800-ACS-2345, 404-3203333
Cancer Information Services
  Tel: 1-800-442-6237

Spain

Fundación Internacional José Carreras, Muntaner, 383 2n.,
  08021 Barcelona
  Fax: 34 93 201 05 88
  e-mail: f.carreras@bcn.servicom.es

2 Frequently used abbreviations

ALL	Acute lymphoblastic leukaemia
AML	Acute myeloid leukaemia
BMT	Bone marrow transplant
CLL	Chronic lymphocytic leukaemia
CML	Chronic myeloid leukaemia
CNS	Central nervous system
DNA	Deoxyribonucleic acid
GVHD	Graft-versus-host disease
PB	Peripheral blood
UK	United Kingdom
USA	United States of America

Index